INTEGRATIVE WELLNESS RULES

A SIMPLE GUIDE TO HEALTHY LIVING

Dr. Jim Nicolai

DIRECTOR OF INTEGRATIVE WELLNESS
AT MIRAVAL RESORT AND SPA

HAY HOUSE

Australia • Canada • Hong Kong • India
South Africa • United Kingdom • United States

First published and distributed in the United Kingdom by:
Hay House UK Ltd, 292B Kensal Rd, London W10 5BE. Tel.: (44) 20 8962 1230;
Fax: (44) 20 8962 1239. www.hayhouse.co.uk

Published and distributed in the United States of America by:
Hay House, Inc., PO Box 5100, Carlsbad, CA 92018-5100. Tel.: (1) 760 431 7695 or
(800) 654 5126; Fax: (1) 760 431 6948 or (800) 650 5115. www.hayhouse.com

Published and distributed in Australia by:
Hay House Australia Ltd, 18/36 Ralph St, Alexandria NSW 2015. Tel.: (61) 2 9669
4299; Fax: (61) 2 9669 4144. www.hayhouse.com.au

Published and distributed in the Republic of South Africa by:
Hay House SA (Pty), Ltd, PO Box 990, Witkoppen 2068. Tel./Fax: (27) 11 467 8904.
www.hayhouse.co.za

Published and distributed in India by:
Hay House Publishers India, Muskaan Complex, Plot No.3, B-2, Vasant Kunj, New
Delhi – 110 070. Tel.: (91) 11 4176 1620; Fax: (91) 11 4176 1630.
www.hayhouse.co.in

Distributed in Canada by:
Raincoast, 9050 Shaughnessy St, Vancouver, BC V6P 6E5. Tel.: (1) 604 323 7100;
Fax: (1) 604 323 2600

The information given in this book should not be treated as a substitute for professional medical advice; always consult a medical practitioner. Any use of information
in this book is at the reader's discretion and risk. Neither the author nor the publisher can be held responsible for any loss, claim or damage arising out of the use, or
misuse, or the suggestions made or the failure to take medical advice.

A catalogue record for this book is available from the British Library.

ISBN 978-1-4019-4049-2

FOR KYLE, JUDE, AVA, AND SARA SUE

CONTENTS

Foreword by Andrew Weil, M.D. ix
Preface xi
Introduction xv

CHECK IN AND DISCOVER

- Decide to Change 3
- Dream Big 5
- Know Your Obstacles 9
- Set Health Goals 13
- Create Positive Rituals 17
- Keep a Journal 19

SUCCESS AND MOTIVATION

- Be Extraordinary 25
- Do Hard Things First 27
- The Law of Threes 31
- The Map and the Mind-Set 35
- Be Proactive 39
- Role Models and Archetypes 41
- Pick a Partner 45
- Take a Day Off 47
- What to Do on Vacation 51

ACCESSING YOUR SPIRITUALITY

- Follow Your Heart 57
- Listen to the Whisper 63
- Believe in Magic 65
- Give the Day to God 69
- Get into Nature 73
- Give to Live 77

YOUR EMOTIONAL HEALTH AND STRESS MANAGEMENT

- Breathe 87
- Go for a Breathwalk 93
- Watch Your Focus 97
- Describe, Investigate, and Evaluate 103
- Swing and a Prayer 107

- Laugh Often. 113
- Find a Friend in a Pet 115
- Turn on Some Tunes. 119

IMPLEMENTING SENSIBLE NUTRITION STRATEGIES
- Eat Right. 125
- Use Olive Oil Abundantly 129
- Eat a Rainbow. 131
- Develop a Taste for Tea. 133
- My Favorite Breakfast 137
- Lay Off the Processed Stuff. 141
- Practice Hari Hachi Bu 143
- "Bate, Bate Chocolate". 145
- Drink More Water. 149

OPTIMIZING VITAMINS, SUPPLEMENTS, AND HERBS
- Optimize Your Vitamin D 155
- Take a Good Daily Multivitamin-Mineral Supplement 159
- Get More Omega-3s. 163
- The Magic of Tulsi 167
- Learn More about 'Shrooms. 171

MANAGING YOUR PHYSICAL BODY
- Walk the Dog 177
- Move Your Body Every Day. 179
- High-Intensity Interval Training 181
- Strength Training 185
- Know Your Trigger Points 191
- My Typical Day. 195

Afterword. 203
Appendixes
- The Anti-Inflammatory Diet. 207
- Dietary Supplements. 215
- A Note on Integrative Medicine. 219

Suggested Reading, Resources, and Products 223
Endnotes 231
Acknowledgments. 243
About the Author 247

FOREWORD

by Andrew Weil, M.D.

I have known the author of this book for more than a decade. Dr. Jim Nicolai was finishing his residency in family medicine when he first came to a workshop I was leading in Tucson, Arizona. Our meeting led him to become one of the first residential fellows at the Arizona Center for Integrative Medicine—a two-year intensive training that gave him the knowledge and skills to practice the kind of medicine I have long taught and practiced. Since he completed the fellowship, he has matured into a highly effective physician. I was delighted when he took the position as the medical director of the integrative wellness center I created at Miraval Resort and Spa.

Practitioners of integrative medicine pay a great deal of attention to lifestyle and to all the factors under our control that influence health and risks of disease. They want to know how their patients eat, how active they are physically, how well they sleep and rest, how they deal with stress, how they use their minds, what they do for fun, how they attend to their spiritual well-being, and more. They are dedicated to promoting health and preventing illness by helping people make better lifestyle choices as well as by offering scientifically informed treatments that emphasize natural, less toxic therapies whenever possible. In order to do this well, physicians must teach by example. They must embody the philosophy and habits they wish to impart to others.

For as long as I've known him, Jim Nicolai has been an inspiring model of health and wellness. He takes very good care of himself and never preaches what he does not practice. Over the years, I've referred many patients to him; he has successfully inspired most of them to make positive changes in their ways of living.

Now he has put his experience into written words to help readers succeed as he has in building and maintaining lifestyles that favor lasting good health. Jim struggles with the same difficulties all of us have: Where do we find motivation to exercise or improve our eating habits? How can we overcome the inertia of being inactive or of eating unconsciously? How do we find time for meditation? In these pages, Jim shares with us the strategies he has used, showing us how to take small steps toward big goals. He writes as he speaks—simply and clearly.

If you were to come to Miraval and have a private consultation with Jim, I know you would come away inspired to take those steps. I believe you can get to know Jim by way of this book and come away with similar inspiration. He has put himself into it, and the voice that comes through is clear, honest, and strong. Listen to it, and let it guide you on the path to wellness.

PREFACE

It's a mouthful to introduce myself as the medical director of the Andrew Weil, M.D., Integrative Wellness Program at Miraval Resort and Spa in Tucson, Arizona. I'd rather describe myself as a health coach. As a physician working in a resort, I often find myself helping people who come to Miraval wanting to change some aspect of their lives. A coach provides motivation and training, and coaching enhances one's positive abilities and actions. Coaching observes subtle distinctions and clarifies the importance and priority of fundamental skills. It is a tool that can show the path to better performance—whether in the things you already do well or things that are challenging for you. A coach is your partner in overcoming obstacles, and he or she will share insights and skills that can move you beyond where you can go on your own. This is what I do. My area of specialty and coaching is integrative health. Let me define what that means.

First of all, let me tell you what health is not. Health really shouldn't be defined as the absence of disease. The definition of disease is the "absence of ease," so explaining something as "the absence of an absence . . ." doesn't seem useful.

My integrative colleagues and I think of health as a wholeness and balance that gives us the resilience to go through the world without being knocked down and staying that way. Health does not imply that we aren't going to get sick or have setbacks, but it does suggest that we can bounce back quickly and regain our balance.

Possessing health allows you to have confidence to walk through the world without dreading its potential dangers. It means you can be exposed to allergens without getting allergies, carcinogens without getting cancer, infectious diseases without getting sick, and stressors without succumbing to stress-related illnesses. Having health also offers a sense of fulfillment and peace that comes with acquiring this level of hardiness and fortitude.

Miraval's Integrative Wellness Program was named purposefully. Health was not mentioned in the title because all of us here wanted wellness to be our focus. While health is the ultimate destination, wellness is the road map that gets you there. I define wellness as the good feeling you get after finding and using a series of personalized, specific strategies that allow you to achieve optimum health. To me, wellness is action just as much as it is a feeling. While health is generalized, wellness is individualized. Strategies might be similar from person to person, but each one carries its unique signature because it matches your personal style.

Practicing integrative medicine enables me to give people these strategies. Integrative medicine is healing oriented as opposed to focusing purely on disease management. It also regards individuals as more than just physical bodies, paying attention to the mental, emotional, spiritual, relational, and even energetic aspects of who they are. When I know a person in this way, I can then devise tools to bring about better balance and wholeness in all of these areas.

Having an understanding of alternative therapies as well as conventional medical methods allows me to select treatments that might be more affordable, less toxic, and *just as* or *more* effective than first using conventional drugs or surgery. If we need conventional methods, fine. It's good to know they are available. It's my job to guide individuals through the maze of confusion and misinformation surrounding which methods to use. My training allows me to discern the good from the bad so I can find the right match of therapies, practices, dietary supplements, and natural remedies, combining them with the best of conventional methods to help you on your journey to health and healing.

Having said that, remember that I don't have all the answers. I don't know everything, but frankly, this idea should be liberating.

First, not having all the answers allows me to continue to be humble. With my ego in check, I realize that I need to continuously search for solutions to keep my health optimized as well as the health of the people I serve. Humility allows me to check out other tools, perspectives, and opinions to find out which ones work for me as well as my clients. If I don't put all the pressure on myself, thinking I have to have all the right answers and can present them in some kind of magical formula, it keeps me vigilant and always looking, and the search itself actually gets to be fun. Unearthing these strategies can become an archaeological adventure—sort of like being Indiana Jones hunting for treasure in the jungle.

Hopefully this explains why you see my homages and references to other authors, trainers, coaches, scholars, doctors, and health practitioners throughout this book—all of whom have added to my set of skills. Finding optimum health is difficult. Doing it on your own seems foolhardy at best. At worst, the demands may create such pressure as to make it completely overwhelming. This can be paralyzing, like Han Solo frozen in carbonite,[1] and I don't want that to happen to me or the people I'm coaching.

Fortunately, I don't have to be an uber-genius or know everything. I just need to use every bit of help I can get along the way. The same goes for you.

This book collects my best strategies to take on that journey.

INTRODUCTION

John Wooden was a legendary basketball player and coach whose UCLA teams won the NCAA championship 10 out of 12 years from 1964 through 1975.[1] They also won 88 games in a row during this span. Coach Wooden carried a $2 bill in his wallet that he never spent. It was a present given to him by his father, Joshua, on his eighth-grade graduation from a school in rural Indiana, given to him so he "would never go broke." Coach Wooden still had the $2 bill when he died on June 4, 2010, at the age of 99. In addition to the money, his dad gave him a three-by-five-inch card that John kept with the $2 bill. On one side of the card was a poem written by Reverend Henry Van Dyke, reminding him of what a man must do to live an honest life. On the other side, his father wrote seven statements as a credo for his son to live by, which went like this:

1. Be true to yourself.

2. Make each day your masterpiece.

3. Help others.

4. Drink deeply from good books—especially the Bible.

5. Make friendship a fine art.

6. Build a shelter against a rainy day.

7. Pray for guidance, and give thanks for your blessings every day.

What a gift of special words, so powerful in their simplicity. I carry these same statements on a three-by-five-inch card in my own wallet out of deep respect and appreciation for John Wooden and his father. Their legacy of wisdom is part of my personal success formula.

This credo made me think about how I practice medicine. As an integrative physician at Miraval, the best advice I can give to guests is usually simple and easy to understand but profound when applied. That kind of advice stuck with me when I learned it from my teachers. It is what I try to put into practice every day, and I coach others to do the same.

Coach Wooden often quoted Mahatma Ghandi when coaching his players: "Learn as if you were to live forever. Live as if you were to die tomorrow." This quote inspires me every day and is at the heart of this book. It is an affirmation, reminding me to continue being passionate while listening to my heart.

This book is a collection of wellness rules I've learned and am sharing in ways that are easy to follow, practical to implement, and effective when put into practice. You can steamroll through all the chapters in a day or go slowly, choosing a couple of pieces that catch your eye or taking one section at a time. "Check In and Discover" shares ideas for listening to yourself and setting goals. These discoveries are built on as you move through the "Success and Motivation" section, where I talk about how it's not knowing what to do that accomplishes our goals; we need help following through and getting them done. "Accessing Your Spirituality" focuses on tapping into the part of you that is connected to something bigger, especially when times get tough. We develop and enhance emotional intelligence in "Your Emotional Health and Stress Management." Next we put all of these pieces to work in everyday routines around "Implementing Sensible Nutrition Strategies," as well as learning about "Optimizing Vitamins, Supplements, and Herbs." Finally, we look at simple approaches to move and keep fit in "Managing Your Physical Body."

Each section is a collection of thoughts, rules, and stories that are meant to inspire, amuse, and give memory cues for your own "Aha!" moments.

I believe these tips will touch you profoundly, as they have me. As you read this book, you might find yourself smiling a bit as you learn, pondering a bit as you think, and moving toward your goals as if there's no tomorrow. You'll find all the inspiration you need to take the time right now and set goals surrounding your health.

Ultimately, I wish for you to discover a more vibrant and fulfilling life by using one, several, or as many of these strategies and concepts as you like—or take them all.

I did.

Here's to your good health,
Dr. Jim

CHECK IN AND DISCOVER

DECIDE
TO CHANGE

The word *decide* comes from the Latin *decidere*, which means "to cut off from." It means to take all of your options, select the one you want, and throw the others out the door.

When people truly decide to do something, it gets done regardless of the obstacles because they have "cut away" any other option from happening. The task, project, or job has become a *must* instead of a *should*. Most of the time we live in a place I like to call "*Should-land.*" Tony Robbins is a personal success coach who often says, "We *should* all over ourselves."

Shoulds usually become *musts* only when the reasons to do something differently are more compelling than staying stuck in familiar and redundant patterns. More often than not, we are frightened into action. A close friend dies suddenly from a heart attack or cancer, and we realize we need to do something about our health *now*. The problem with fear is that it goes away with time, and if that's our only reason to change, it usually doesn't stick.

With that said, my questions to anyone reading this book are: *Do you really want to change? And if so, why? Outside of fear, what are five reasons why you absolutely have to change right now?*

Talk about this with a friend, partner, mentor, or someone else you trust. Try to convince him or her why you need to do this. See if he or she believes you.

If that person does, read on. If not, all this book will offer is yet again more of the same information you've read before; maybe a bit of entertainment but nothing that will take you to the next level.

That is up to you.

DREAM BIG

What do you want? Most of us have forgotten how to dream outside of our sleeping world. For some reason, the little kid in us—the one who has no problem suspending reality in favor of Fantasy Island—has gone to sleep.

Maybe it's because all of our dreams have been shot down in favor of the practicalities of making a living and putting food on the table. Maybe we're afraid to step out and take a chance to think of a world filled with unlimited possibilities. Reasons abound to justify why we don't dream. All of my mentors and heroes are dreamers. If they can do it, why can't I?

Steven Pressfield has written one of my favorite books called *Gates of Fire.*[1] It is about the ancient Battle of Thermopylae, which was made famous by the movie *300.* He has recently written a series of nonfiction books about defeating resistance and living the life we were meant for. In one of these books, called *Do the Work!,* he says, "A child has no trouble believing the unbelievable, nor does the genius or the madman. It's only you and I, with our big brains and our tiny hearts, who doubt and overthink and hesitate."[2]

It's time for us to think about our dreams for a change. It's time for us to dream big. I often invite people to form an image of what optimum health might look like for them or imagine what their ideal self might be with all of their obstacles eliminated. I ask them to tell me some of the deepest desires of their heart—what keeps coming up for them to do, be, say, or live that may not be happening yet.

A guest I saw at Miraval is an interventional cardiologist practicing in the Midwest. She doesn't really want to practice medicine in the way she does now; in fact, she hates what she does. It's eating her alive. She has every stress-related problem you can think of, from headaches and gastritis to insomnia and palpitations. What she would really love to do is work with horses and handicapped kids.

After we talked, I discovered that she lives very close to where I used to live and practice. And isn't it interesting—I know someone in that community who has a ranch with horses and engages with disabled little ones to build balance, muscle tone, and self-esteem.

I believe this is how life works. There's a force out there that wants us to live our dreams. We just have to get over, under, or through all of the walls we create. Anne Parker, a colleague of mine at Miraval, says, "Change happens when the discomfort of the familiar outweighs the fear of the unknown." That is so true.

I gave this individual the contact information for the ranch. I hope she acts on this bit of synchronicity; I don't believe in accidents. Stuff happens for a reason . . . all of it. I may not be able to see or feel the connections in the moment—and I may never see them—but they are always there.

My first recommendation for her was to start dreaming big. I asked her to make a vision board—a piece of poster board with cut-out pictures, words, phrases, and ideas from magazines, newspapers, and paper advertisements that describe the desires of your heart or your ideal self. I suggest you make one, too. Design your vision board by taking the dreams of your imagination and making them concrete—even if they're just pictures on a poster board. One time, my wife cut out a picture of the figure she wanted, pasted it in her journal, cut off the head, and put her own face on the empty space. I once cut out the picture of the six-pack abdominal muscles I wanted to have. I kept thinking about what I would look like with abs like that. It took me 12 weeks and some serious sweat, but I got them—and the vision in my head kept me motivated to make it happen. Transformation occurs from the inside out.

Anything you desire to change on the outside must first be changed internally. The physical transformation happens later. Start by dreaming it up. Seeing the vision inside is the most important part and has to happen first.

As you create a goal, first understand what the destination looks like in your mind. Using all of your senses, flesh out every aspect of what will happen in your imagination. How does it look, smell, and taste? What sounds do you hear? What do you hear people saying? What do you say when you've made it? How does it make you feel to have made your dream come true?

Make this vision real by putting it plainly in front of you every single day. Then work on the next big question: *What's getting in the way?*

KNOW YOUR OBSTACLES

Lou Holtz is a former football coach of Notre Dame, and the last person to coach their football team to a national championship.

In his book *Winning Every Day,* he describes a typical conversation he would have with his team members every year before the season started. He explained to them that there would be certain obstacles the team would have to face—an injury to one or more star players, an illness, suspension, or some other turn of events that would reduce their chances of having a successful season. He would tell the team that these obstacles were not imaginary; they would definitely happen. Obstacles would come no matter what; it was just a matter of what shape they would take. With that in mind, he would then challenge his team to come together to find a way to overcome whatever obstacles would present themselves throughout the season.

He warned them how foolish it was to think that problems would not arise. More important, he fixed their mind-set on the goal and the solution, not on what would get in the way.

It's not a question of whether obstacles are going to come. They will. The question is, What are you going to do about it? How will you get over, under, or through any wall that impedes your journey to accomplish your goals for health and living optimally?

With this in mind, it is important to at least be clear on what's currently impeding your progress. Write down on a piece of paper what limitations you might have. What negative patterns of behavior do you need to change that seem to stop or stall your best attempts at transforming your life? What people may be sabotaging your quest for improvement? Write all this down.

Clarity is powerful in that it can help you recognize ongoing patterns that work against achieving your objective. The more you understand what's in the way of getting where you want to go, the better you can figure out how to get from here to there.

How you see yourself is important. Getting feedback from mentors and friends you trust and who are willing to offer proactive criticism may allow you to see things you may not be aware of, but be careful with this. As you are getting started, allow yourself small doses of this kind of critique. Let people give you criticism in the "reverse Oreo" way: two bits of good words, the cream on the outside, sandwiched between one piece of hard critical darkness.

Once you know what you want and what's in the way, the next step is to figure out the plan (strategies) to get you where you want to go. This is what I call bridging the gap. You want to create a tactical action plan of simple steps to begin the process.

Many people may know what they need to do, but the act of doing it—the application of that knowledge—somehow gets lost in the shuffle.

This is when we need strategies that are simple and doable— meaning we can somehow fit them into our schedule and get them done. They may even be fun.

The tips in the upcoming pages will help you begin to select a set of strategies and action steps that take you toward your ideal self, the health that you deserve, and the life you need to live.

Good luck.

SET HEALTH GOALS

Most of us set goals in our professional lives: be vice president of the company in ten years, make our first million by age 40, sell 50,000 cubits by first quarter's end, and so on. Why is it that we don't apply the same strategy to our health?

Whenever I'm talking to a guest about designing health goals, I bring up the SMART method.[1] Goals are written in the form of future accomplishments that allow you to continually grow and expand. Following this formula can help make your goals clear, concise, and easy to follow.

A SMART goal is one that is specific, measurable, attainable, relevant, and has a time frame. For a goal to be accomplished, it cannot be described in generalities. You do not want to lose weight; you want to lose 20 pounds of body fat over 16 weeks. Being specific allows you to know exactly what your target is, how to quantify both the endpoint and your progress along the way, whether it can realistically be achieved, and by when you need it to be done.

Your goals should be believable and attainable but should also stretch you a bit. Your goal should be nothing too drastic but just a bit out of your comfort zone.

Relevance is all about not being tempted to do something because it sounds great or seems easy to do but because it speaks to your personal vision and mission of life, both in the short and long-term.

Setting a time frame to your goals locks them into reality. Now you have a deadline. Simply deciding when you will achieve something can inspire and motivate you to change.

Some final notes on goals: I like to add two more letters and make it the SMART-TV method. I think goals should also have what Tony Robbins calls the "right TV" or *transformational vocabulary.*[2] Goals are designed to set a clear target in front of you; using words that get you to that target are essential. Note the following example:

I want to lose 15 pounds in 12 weeks.

This has all the requirements of the SMART goal, right? Notice how this next one is different:

I will lose 15 pounds in 12 weeks while thoroughly enjoying the process!

Words are powerful; they can set our focus and motivate us, or they can drag us down. When I think my goal is hard work or drudgery, I have to force myself through the changes. But what if I make the process entertaining? That sets up a whole different set of rules that may give me a better chance of getting it done. Choose your words carefully.

Goals also need to be written down, preferably signed and dated by you and an accountability partner, whomever that may be (see "Pick a Partner").

You should review your goals at least twice daily. The reason why we don't accomplish our goals is that we forget about them. We have too many things going on in our busy lives, and when we don't check in on our progress, we neglect our action plan. We are either growing or dying; there is no in between.

I suggest putting your goals in the front page of your journal or on the outside of the kitchen refrigerator or both, for that matter. The more access you have to your goals and your action strategy, the more they are on your mind. The more they are on your mind, the more you can accomplish them.

CREATE POSITIVE RITUALS

My friend and colleague at Miraval, Leigh Weinrub, is a tennis coach and wellness counselor. She talks to her clients about creating positive daily rituals as a way to guide oneself toward health.

I agree with her.

Athletes do this all the time—creating rituals. Look at a baseball player as he gets into the batter's box: he adjusts the gloves, kicks his cleats, plants his feet, takes a couple of practice swings, and then he is ready to go. Examine the tennis pro as she serves or the golfer on the putting green: they repeat the same motions to do what they do. The basketball player shooting free throws looks something like this: right foot on the line, bounce the ball three times, spin it, take a deep breath, and then shoot, staying up on the toes.

Athletes do these rituals over and over again until they can do them in their sleep.

Rituals involve creating patterns and then doing them repeatedly until they become part of your identity. You don't have to think to do it; you just begin the process and let it take you on your way. It's no wonder we have a hard time letting go of bad habits—they are negative rituals that have become part of us.

Health and beauty strategies should be included in our rituals. They can become habitual if we let them. We should find a way to do them frequently until they become part of us.

The hard part is always beginning.

It involves a bit of creativity to start the process and make it your own. Oftentimes someone will teach you certain actions to perform. That's my job, whether it's breathing techniques, taking supplements, exercising, or making proper food choices. Ultimately it's up to you to find the right time and place to do them.

Then come the repetitions, what we call the mother of skill, which grind the action into habit. Habit becomes ritual when it incorporates ceremony and a reverence for the power of what those actions bring about. Good rituals are meaningful and fulfilling and induce feelings of pride and accountability.

We are living our truth.

And more to the point, we usually know when we are in the midst of a bad habit that's got to change. Isn't it interesting that the momentum of repetition creates patterns that are hard to stop? Whether it's the glass of wine that turns into three or that evening bowl of ice cream, the incessant shopping for meaningless items, too many cups of coffee, or working our bodies into the ground—we can usually spot a bad habit.

The challenge is can we do something about it?

Naming the problem is key. Usually sharing this with another individual who wants to help support us is the next step. Then comes a whole lot of hard work.

Remember, repetition and momentum can work for us if we let them.

We just have to start the ball rolling, put our heads down, and keep moving forward.

⁎

KEEP A JOURNAL

If it's worth living, it's worth recording.[1]

Those words have stayed in my memory. They've been my motivation for keeping a journal since my early 20s. Journals have been living scrapbooks for everything I've done. From ticket stubs of favorite movies, concerts, and plays to articles found in papers or magazines; pictures of my wife, Sara, and the kids; works of art from the little ones; snapshots from friends and family; brainstorming ideas and dreams; goals—signed and dated; actions items for the upcoming day . . . I keep all of these in my journal.

I also try to make an entry at least every few days as a running commentary on what's going on in my life. It could be what's up with the news, weather, and sports of the day; my reaction to a particular event or situation; or an inspiring idea or memory I want to capture. If it pops into my head, it goes down on paper. Some of these have been real gems.

I also find it fascinating to look at my past journals. They are stored in a large wooden chest. It's amazing to see what was going on way back when, what I was thinking, who was in my life at the time, and how I was responding to things, especially from a reference point of where I am today.

My journals provide a healthy dose of perspective, knowing where I am and from where I've come. All those tragedies I thought were so devastating don't seem as bad; and all of those victories that I thought were fantastic were good but not so tremendous.

Life seems more intriguing when taken from this vantage point.

It gives me a sense of calm that I turned out all right throughout the twists and turns of life. Journaling helps to frame the world around me as I am going through it, knowing that there's a lot going on at a rapid pace but that I'm also a meaningful part of that journey. And ultimately, it gives me satisfaction to know that I'm still here putting the puzzle pieces of my life together—that they have formed a particular picture but there's still more to go.

I liken it to a photo mosaic, where a larger image is made out of hundreds or thousands of tinier pictures. As I record my life, a picture begins to develop, and it adds to all the other reflections I've put together to ultimately coalesce into something greater. What eventually appears may take months or years to see, but as I look back on journal after journal, I begin to notice patterns, and eventually a grander picture of me and where I am on my journey forms. It gives me a reference point to keep moving in a desired direction or to take a step back and go somewhere else.

My journals keep me excited as a collector of memories and experiences to see what adventures may be lurking around the corner and what bigger picture I might be creating. There's nothing better than finishing one book only to open up another.

And somewhere down the road, I know I will feel a sense of satisfaction that I have left a legacy of my life through these journals. It may be my children or their children who might want to know a bit more about their grandfather, and all they will have to do is open the wooden chest. My oldest son just finished an essay about his great-grandfather, who was an Army Corps Engineer in the First World War.

He built roads and bridges in France, and as he interviewed my father-in law, we were getting to know someone who lived through two world wars and the Great Depression. We saw his old leather army bag with the measuring tape he used to gauge the length of whatever he was building. I saw his old holster; it had been to Belgium and back. Having a link to that time through this man was an amazing feeling. I wish I had been able to read some of his letters; it would have taken me to that time and place but also deeper into the man who was living through it.

That's what I want my journals to be as well. It's a gift to those who want to learn about me and the life I've lived.

As a writer and a lover of books, I personally love the feeling of holding a pen in my hand and writing on paper. You need to choose your own favorite way to journal. The only important thing is that you get it down. Write a blog and update it regularly. Talk into a recorder. Use a smartphone or iPad. Keep a scrapbook or a collection of photos, videos, and family movies. Anything you can do to record your life can bring remarkable clarity to your journey.

If it's worth living, it's worth recording!

Once you dream up your vision, the biggest challenge is always taking the first step. The fact that you may not know how to get to your ultimate destination is irrelevant; getting a move on is what's important. Now that you have started with journal in hand, a tangible dream to move toward, your target clarified, and your goals specified, it's time to learn tips to keep you on track, especially when the obstacles of resistance want to knock you off.

SUCCESS AND MOTIVATION

BE
EXTRAORDINARY

When you take the word *extraordinary* apart, it simply means more than ordinary. To be better than ordinary, the question comes down to math. *How much* more than ordinary do we need to be to see results?

Put your thumb and forefinger about an inch apart—that's how much. Just a bit more than ordinary is what we need to see change. Some of my colleagues call this the "extra 5 percent" or the "two-degree difference." I like to show it with my fingers—just *this much.*

The trick is consistency. It's not the doing extra that counts. Most of us do that. It's doing it over and over without fail, whether we like it or not. That's when results come.

The challenge is that you may not see much in the realm of results during the first few weeks or months. A two-degree difference over two weeks seems tiny and certainly not worth the effort required. But project that two-degree difference over six months, a couple of years, or a decade, and you've taken a completely different direction in your life. Your journey has a new trajectory and, consequently, a different destination.

It doesn't have to be big changes. The best ones are usually small and simple to do—like practicing breathing techniques, drinking more water, feeling and expressing gratitude, walking, and praying.

Done regularly, they can change your life.

DO HARD
THINGS FIRST

I had to deal with this issue on a personal level one morning as I woke to the bleating of my wife's alarm. There is nothing worse than being blasted awake by the high-pitched shriek of an electronic device, especially at 4:30 in the morning. My problem was that the clock wasn't on my side of the bed, so I couldn't smash it.

Being a morning person, I can usually get up without an alarm. My wife, Sara, on the other hand, is not blessed with this particular skill. She normally loves to sleep in and would willingly do so any chance she can get. This morning would not be one of those times. A wake-up call was required.

Sara is a very good nurse. She started doing "sanity shifts" back at the hospital when our kids got old enough to go to school. The only work she could get during this time had her starting at the surgery center bright and early at 6 A.M.; so much for sleeping in. The episode with the alarm was to be one of her first shifts. Unfortunately, I had not yet gotten used to her getting up before me, let alone at 4:30 in the morning—a stretch for anyone, even a morning person.

So on this particular morning, I found myself awake at 4:30 and faced with a dilemma: unless I could get to the gym before Sara left at 5:30, I wouldn't get to work out that day.

Now you have to understand something critical to my health. Getting to the gym in the morning is a priority. Morning exercise is not only important, but it also has become part of my identity. It is just as much a part of who I am as it is what I do. I needed to get to the gym. As a result, I was faced with a distinct challenge. For the first time in a while (Sara had been home with the kids for at least a couple of years), I had to figure out if I could motivate myself to get going so early and get back home in time before she left for work. Fortunately, the fitness center where I exercise is five minutes away, so distance wasn't an issue.

It was just a matter of me deciding to get to the gym now or later. Did I get it done first thing, or would I find some space later in the day to get around to it? Personally, exercise is something I enjoy, but the windows of opportunity have shrunk as my responsibilities at work and home have increased. The challenge is obviously figuring out when I can get it done.

This situation got me thinking about the concept of doing hard things first.

Anytime I am faced with a decision about when to do something, chances are I need to do it now. Sooner is better than later. This has become a discipline learned after hours of excuses, stalling, distractions, and ultimately, doing nothing.

Especially when effort is involved, if I find myself postponing the activity I know I need to do for any length of time beyond 5 to 15 minutes, it usually doesn't get accomplished. Something bigger and better comes along to divert my attention; something comes up that takes more time than I thought, or I find myself looking at the clock, it's late in the day, and I'm just too damn tired, apathetic, or overwhelmed to make it happen.

Doing hard things first is all about making sure you accomplish your most challenging activity as soon as possible. If whatever you are trying to do seems difficult or demanding—if there is resistance behind it and you think you may not get this activity done for whatever reason—then make sure you check it off your list the first chance you get.

I do my hardest things in the morning. It makes me feel great to know that my biggest accomplishment has been taken care of early in the day. I feel good that I have been accountable to myself. I start the day with positive momentum, and it seems like the rest of my to-dos are easier as I begin my day in the right frame of mind.

Doing hard things first has saved me in so many ways. Use it to help you get your most difficult challenges accomplished.

It's all downhill from there.

THE LAW
OF THREES

When I first began my integrative practice, I would see patients for two hours and then have them return the following week to receive a treatment plan. During the seven days between visits, I would research their conditions, ponder over what recommendations to make, and then type up a set of instructions—often several pages long—describing the best integrative approaches to follow.

I felt proud of myself for doing this. Most doctors don't write prescriptions like these. Some of them seemed like books—novellas at least. I could tell that my patients were a bit surprised when they saw such a plan, often encased in a large folder or binder.

Ultimately, I got the impression that this kind of treatment plan wasn't so much about them as it was about me. The feeling I was getting from patients was that they appreciated the wealth of information, but in all honesty, it was just too much.

So I scrapped it.

Then I happened upon the Law of Threes, and it changed how I practice completely.

The Law of Threes suggests that whenever we are faced with change, less is more. Small steps are much more practical than huge changes. It's better to stack little pieces of improvement on top of each other incrementally over time, and the only way you do this is to think that you can. Overwhelming feelings crash down on the person who feels unsure or unable, so start small and doable.

The Law of Threes says that when we are implementing change, we can think of three things to do. We can get our heads around three action steps, especially when they are small and not too crazy and we think we can get them done. One, two, three is doable. Four is too many—seriously. Not only is one more than three too many, but chances are it will be so overwhelming that either heads explode (messy), or you will find yourself unable to do the first three things because you've piled too much on.

This may seem ridiculous, but I can tell you it has happened so often in my practice that I am actually afraid when I give a fourth suggestion. Whether this has been studied or not, I don't know, but I'm telling you, it's true.

Now the brilliant thing about your mind is that I can give you three categories to focus on and place two or three things underneath each without you feeling dazed or confused. The minute I add a fourth, we are both finished.

In my practice at Miraval, I will often categorize my suggestions into three headings: *stuff to take, stuff to do,* and *people to see.* (I don't like using big medical words; it never helps.) For instance, I will give someone three supplements and herbs to try, three action steps to focus on, and three of my best experts, guides, or practitioners to experience. This approach focuses on the basics. At Miraval, the guests who see me feel that what I give them fits their situations and their personalities, is simple enough for them to do, and can be done right now.

If they leave with just this bit of change moving in the right direction, it may be what it takes to change their lives. I'm not looking for big change—just two or three degrees or 5 percent sustained over time (see "Be Extraordinary"). My goal is to get people started with the belief that this is how change works. Their job is to suspend judgment, put their heads down, and work the program for the next 12 weeks. If the change sticks, then we're onto something.

Remember, positive change starts with three things—never four.

THE MAP AND
THE MIND-SET

The biggest challenge to dreaming big is the fear and doubt that creep up when we don't know how to get there. Achieving our goals can seem distant, and when we don't know how to arrive at the destination, we may find ourselves starting to panic, feeling unworthy or incapable of the journey.

We need to understand that most innovators and inventors didn't know exactly how to get to their vision before they started moving toward it. Thomas Edison said, "I will not say I failed 1,000 times, I will say that I discovered there are 1,000 ways that can cause failure."[1]

Not knowing how doesn't mean standing still.

What we need is a proper map and mind-set. Having the right map helps us navigate so we don't move aimlessly. It guides us in the right general direction as we take steps toward our goals. The right mind-set is an attitude that says, "I'm getting there no matter what," even if we seem lost. As we discover that a process isn't working, a good mind-set reminds us to take a step back, figure out another way, and start moving again.

Laying the groundwork with concepts like being extraordinary and doing hard things first sets the stage for the map—or the major action plan—that comes with a disciplined mind-set. We make the map each day. It comes from knowing our larger goals, usually attainable 12 to 16 weeks into the future. I like three months.

With that in mind, we set time aside each day to decide what three to five small things to do to get us one step closer to our destination. This is the map. The first one or two actions steps should be the harder ones for us to accomplish; this is practicing hard things first. It may be something like the following.

- Wake up at 5:00 A.M. and get to the gym, do a 20-minute high-intensity aerobic workout I call HIIT (High-Intensity Interval Training—I explain this in a later chapter).

- Go for a walking meditation called breathwalking (also in an upcoming chapter), along with a morning prayer.

- Take your supplements.

I note this in my journal every morning under the title "To Do Today."

My three-month goals are usually written on the first page of my journal, along with the reasons why I am doing them. Then every day I practice being extraordinary by getting at least three things done in the direction of my goals (remember, I like *threes*).

My mind-set keeps me looking at my goals every day, understanding why I am working on them, visualizing what it will feel like to accomplish them, and expressing gratitude for getting them done. I review my vision board, look to my role models, and focus on the journey—not the destination.

What keeps my map easy to follow is a practical philosophy of getting things done that seems so simple but has been a major "Aha!"

personally. It is the concept of accomplishing my goals in *no extra time*—what I call NET[2] activity.

I love this concept. It's obvious that most of us don't have a whole lot of extra time to do other things. I'm usually spinning a fair amount of plates in my life on a regular basis, just like most of the guests who come and see me at Miraval. Wouldn't it be novel to think about doing things within our busy lives—in no extra time—as opposed to lopping it all together with all the other things we've got going on? It certainly throws the "I don't have time for that" excuse out the window.

The notion of NET isn't mine; it was created by Tony Robbins. I wish I could claim it. Fortunately, I'm in the business of helping people find strategies that work and not worrying about from where they came. This one works; it's brilliant and profound at the same time. Essentially it means to take all of the things you already spend time doing and insert an action into them. How much time do you spend driving, walking, working out, or watching television? Why not link a healthy action to each of these activities so that whenever you do them, the healthy choice follows? For example, I do breathing exercises in the car and while walking my dog. I read motivational books or listen to inspiring music and messages while riding a stationary bike. The biofeedback tool I teach at Miraval is something I do after lunch while I'm at my computer. Can you respond to e-mails while walking on a treadmill?

If Mr. Robbins can, so can you.

For every healthy choice I am trying to add to an individual's repertoire, invariably the ones that work best fit into NET.

Give it a try.

BE PROACTIVE

Our mental chatter gets us in trouble.

The random dialogue in my head is usually an ongoing mish-mash of thought categories that range from the interesting and wonderful all the way to the weird and confusing. At times I have a hard time shutting off the noise. How about you?

The human brain is an awesome computer. Among other things, it's specially designed to answer any question that comes to us, no matter how random, bizarre, or complex.

Problems occur when we ask the wrong questions.

The minute I ask my brain something like, *Why does this always happen to me?* or *Why can't I ever get it right?* I get answers like, "Because you deserve it" or "Since you're a nimrod."

Ask a stupid question and you know what you get. . . .

The questions I should be asking the computer in my brain are ones that can help me find solutions, not ones that sabotage my efforts.

Show me instead of *why* me.

I like asking the following proactive questions when I'm in a pickle:

- *How can I use this?*

- *Where's the lesson here?*

- *How can I de-stress the situation?*

- *What's the next right thing to do?*

- *Help, please [as I look up to the sky].*

- *Is this [feeling, thought, reaction] working for me? If not, what's a different way?*

It can be so easy to focus on questions that aren't helpful or don't work. I'd rather have my noggin help me reach my ultimate destination, not hinder me. Asking proactive questions moves me in the direction of my goals.

So, be sure to feed your mind the right riddles.

ROLE
MODELS AND
ARCHETYPES

I love movies. I'm wired so that when I see a film, I'm instantly transported. The characters, the setting, the cinematography, and the mood take me very quickly into that imaginary world where, for the next couple of hours, it's hard to get out of. This is great when the movie is a good one, not so good when it's garbage.

My favorite movies usually involve mythical archetypes and themes. Films like *The Lord of the Rings* trilogy, *Star Wars,* the *Indiana Jones* or *Harry Potter* series, *Avatar,* and old greats like *Casablanca* speak to me in ways that are hard to explain.

They all involve what Joseph Campbell calls the Hero's Journey,[1] the timeless story of a man or woman coming of age. The path of the hero winds its way through an array of twists and turns that starts with the call, where our hero first learns of his destiny. Typically this call to adventure seems too much to bear. It's messy, complex, and overwhelming; it brings up fear, insecurity, or a sense of inadequacy and ultimately refusal to heed the call. The refusal more often than not brings about the road of trials, otherwise known as the initiation or what I would call the apprenticeship.

Your destiny isn't going away anytime soon, however. You signed up for it, even if the world says you didn't.

The good thing for you is that help is on the way—usually in the guise of a mentor (think Yoda, Obi-Wan, Gandalf, Dumbledore, Neytiri) guiding you along your adventure. This is the point where you accept your destiny and cross the threshold between an ordinary life and the life of your dreams. You leave the familiar and enter a world of uncertainty and danger, where all that you know is gone.

Some call this moment the belly of the whale. This is the point when you enter your darkest hour; however, this low point really symbolizes the death of your old self. There is grief, but by entering this place, you demonstrate a willingness to transform from your old self into the new.

As you enter the road of trials, you encounter new and strange worlds where you will be tested; you will learn, grow, and be tested again. Enemies and allies will be encountered, and ultimately you will come face-to-face with your greatest challenge.

Think of Luke Skywalker in the cave facing the Darth Vader that is ultimately himself. This crisis or series of ordeals is where heroes face their greatest fear, risking their lives to be transformed by responding heroically.

And because of this, the hero is changed forever, committed to using his new self in a different way. He is rewarded (usually with gifts or recognition) and chooses to use these gifts to go back to the ordinary world, where he can serve, protect, defend, and teach a new way to those who will receive it and be changed in turn.

I love these stories. They remind me of my own personal journey. Yes, I feel like I am meant for something bigger than a humdrum existence. Don't you?

Watching these powerful movies prompts me to remember my destiny and work toward fulfilling it. They retell the story and inspire me to manage my fear and realize that the unknown is my friend—that I do have helpers, seen and unseen, and will learn something on the road that changes everything, bringing me one step closer to my dreams.

And so I collect things: mementoes, memorabilia, posters, movie props, and so on. I have a huge statue of Indiana Jones holding the golden idol after the opening scene in *Raiders of the Lost Ark*. It tells me to keep seeking—to be an archaeologist for more healing tips. Another statue of Luke and Yoda from *The Empire Strikes Back* reminds me of the training I need. A smaller statue of Captain Kirk prompts me to take risks if I'm going to sit in the captain's chair. A letter opener with a Spartan shield and sword from the movie *300* keeps me fighting for my beliefs. Wands from the *Harry Potter* movies symbolize the ongoing battle between good and evil.

The biggest challenge, I think, is that it can be so easy to forget my mission. The current of life can take me over and lull me into the sleep of a complacent world. Anything that brings me back to the journey I'm taking and challenges me to be the hero I'm supposed to be reminds me to be vigilant. Vigilance is key.

PICK A PARTNER

Modeling is one of the secrets of change.

If you want to achieve success in anything, find people who have already succeeded in that category and model their behavior. Discover how they use their minds—thoughts and feelings—and their bodies to produce the results you want.

One of the best ways to unlearn old habits and develop newer, healthier ones is to spend time with people who have the habits you want—to model them. Your choice of friends and acquaintances is a powerful influence on your behavior. All too often the people we hang out with are sabotaging our healthy behavior instead of encouraging it or keeping us accountable.

If you want to change your eating habits, spend more time with people who eat healthier than you do. If you want to exercise more, keep company with people who not only work out but also enjoy the process. If you want to better manage stress, find an emotionally intelligent partner who handles stressful situations well.

Besides, it's nice to have someone you trust who can help remind you of your dreams and goals.

The journey to wellness is much more satisfying when it's shared.

TAKE A DAY OFF

I learned this from Bill Phillips and his Body for Life program.[1] There is something magical about taking a day off from my vigilance— whether that is the strictness of my diet and exercise program, my meditation practice, my daily writing . . . whatever. One day weekly, I allow myself to be completely free from the discipline of most of my wellness strategies. If I want to have a bacon double cheeseburger with fries and a soda from the local fast-food restaurant, so be it. If I want to take a nap in the middle of the day, fine. Popcorn at the movies—fair enough. Whatever I can possibly imagine—even a fried Mars bars with bacon—is on the list.

This does a number of positive things for me.

First, it gives me a break. It takes serious energy to say no all the time; going against the mainstream current of life requires a fair amount of restraint. Every so often, it is nice to loosen my grip when I'm holding on tightly.

Especially with food and drink, if I can save all of the cravings I might have during the week, knowing that for one day, I can have whatever I want, certain cravings begin to fade or disappear entirely when I actually have permission to indulge in them. As for the cravings that stick with me, the feeding frenzy is on. This works because I have given myself the right to do so.

The minute I tell a Miraval guest that his or her unseemly behavior is forever banned, it usually marks the start of an obsession that culminates in the complete overindulgence of whatever action I wanted to extinguish. When I tell you that French fries are off limits, you suddenly can't get those greasy potatoes off your mind. A big helping of cheesy fries finds its way into your gullet, and more important, after the guilt and the shame of your mishap, you feel so bad about yourself that you realize you're not meant for this healthy stuff, you will always be a fat slob, and you might as well move on to pizza and eat yourself into oblivion. That's so stupid, but we do it all the time.

All I know is that for me, a couple of things happen when I take a day off. Eating so well for six days in a row allows me to discover just how wonderful food can make me feel. When you suddenly do the exact opposite, it doesn't take long before you feel like absolute garbage. My days off are usually on Sundays. The minute I wake up on Monday morning feeling like I need to brush the hair off my teeth and immediately go into detox is the exact time I recommit to my healthy eating plan. This kind of negative reinforcement keeps me determined to stay on the program. I can't afford to feel that badly any longer than a couple of hours—yuck.

More to the point, having the permission to do whatever I want one day a week keeps me motivated because I don't feel like I'm stuck in a lifestyle prison for the rest of my life. I don't have to feel bad about having cravings, but I also don't have to indulge them the minute they cross my mind. I can manage these impulses under my rules and with a sense of control I didn't have beforehand.

From a scientific standpoint, it is also beneficial to periodically give the body a signal that it isn't starving, especially when one is regularly limiting calories while doing intense exercise. Whenever you begin to burn large quantities of fat, genetic messages, biochemical signals, and metabolic processes warn that the famine may be just around the corner. Periodically overfeeding gives the body a message that everything is okay.

I think this works for any behavior, regardless of what and how we put things in our mouths. Give it a try.

I would also caution those individuals who have a tendency to binge or be compulsive in their behaviors. If this is you—and you know who you are—go slowly. Give yourself one meal or a couple of hours of permitted indulgence. Allow yourself some autonomy to make choices for yourself. See if giving yourself this element of freedom works to keep you on course.

It works for me.

WHAT TO DO ON VACATION

Along with the concept of taking a day off, it's important to think about what we do when we let down our guard.

Vacations can sometimes be very tough on health. They are sort of surreal, and if we're not careful, they can offer us an excuse to binge on food, drink, and inactivity in such a way that we may not be able to recover from it. I don't want vacations to bring about a tailspin that's too hard to pull out of; I need to be able to have fun but still manage my life in a healthy fashion.

For me, vacation is often just another place I go with my wife and kids as I follow them on their adventures. Outside of activities with them, there are small windows of opportunity to get away, get quiet, or go on a date with my sweetie. It's kind of like home; if you don't seize the opportunities you have, you lose them. I don't know if vacation is any less stressful than life at home; it's just in a different location.

We often travel with other families when we go on holiday. I find that sometimes our friends may not have the same conceptions of health or healthy behaviors as we do. Wanting to enjoy my time with these folks, I may have to pick and choose my battles around the health choices that are most important to me.

I often have to let some of these go, and truth be told, sometimes I find myself easily slipping into bad behaviors that I might have done in the past but don't do now. Darn it.

Have you ever gone back to your hometown where you grew up or spent time with family and found yourself falling into similar patterns of what you did when you were younger?

Whether it's the food I eat, the moods I get into, how people treat me, or reactions I have in response to that treatment—all of it seems quite different when I go back home as compared to what my normal routine is outside of family and friends. I fall back into similar patterns quicker than I might think.

This is something I need to guard against.

My proactive response to vacation is to pick some behaviors that I will absolutely maintain—whether it's my exercise routine (or some variation to it), some dietary choices like eating a good breakfast every day, going on my morning walks, or prayer time. If I'm really watching things, I might also pick a couple of negative patterns I want to try to put a leash on—things like drinking too much caffeine or alcohol, staying up too late, forgetting about my meditative breathing, or not taking my vitamins.

And then I let the rest go.

I think that's the key. It's kind of like "what happens in Vegas stays in Vegas." I try to enjoy myself, spend time with people who make me laugh, limit time with those who rub me the wrong way, and play as often as possible with my little ones and others whose company I appreciate. I try to stay mindful of how my body is responding on vacation and write in my journal most days. It helps me to document the trip and take notes on what's going on with my life, my relationships, and ultimately my health.

The first and most important thing to do when I get home from vacation is to plan for the next day to be just like my normal routine, even if I have to fight a bit harder to make it happen.

Momentum is a tricky thing. Bad behavior can build a rhythm just as much as good behavior. I want to break the pattern from vacation as soon as I can if I have strung together a chain of poor choices. Consequently, the most important response to what I do over the holidays or after a trip has to do with my choices when the party is over. If I can get back into my normal routine over the first three days of returning from a family vacation, then I'm usually good. What I do during the first week back is critical.

It's not vacation that trips us up; it's the bad momentum created by living in holiday mode and the poor choices that follow. I don't want that kind of noose around my neck. I may let my guard down a bit on vacation, but I am vigilant to jump right back into my healthy rituals the minute I get back.

Back from vacation with motivation strategies in hand, moving forward despite obstacles and resistance, remember that health is not just the actions you commit to. It's also wholeness and balance.

We are whole persons—physical bodies, of course, but also mental, emotional, and spiritual beings. Having access to the part of us that is connected to something bigger and broader is just as important as eating right and exercising. The following section offers tools to point you in the direction of greater spiritual health.

ACCESSING YOUR SPIRITUALITY

FOLLOW
YOUR HEART

This phrase is metaphorical.

What do we mean when we say it?

Are we really referring to the muscle in the center of our chest that pumps blood? Is that what we should follow? Probably not, and yet, scientifically, we have discovered new insights about how the heart works that may motivate us to do exactly that.

I lead a workshop at Miraval called Finding the Zone that is near and dear to my heart (pun intended). It comes from my work and affiliation with a company called HeartMath. For the past 20 years, they have been on the leading edge of identifying new technology to manage emotional states and optimize performance by utilizing the power of heart intelligence.

Four thousand years ago, ancient philosophers and physicians in India and the Middle East spoke of the heart as a bridge between mind and soul. Traditional Chinese physicians thought that blood vessels were the channels by which the heart distributed this information. Ancient Hindu texts explained the heart to be the fulcrum between an individual and the cosmos. Every spiritual tradition has claimed the heart to be the centerpiece and guidepost to a way of living that brings further enlightenment and fulfillment. That's pretty heavy stuff. This idea continues to be propagated in so many poems, plays, songs, and operas—with or without soap—that we come across every day.

The disconnect of thinking about the heart as purely a mechanical organ and nothing else came about 300 years ago, when we started cutting up the body and looking inside. What we saw was this tiny muscle that pumps blood. Physicians of that day were probably expecting more than that—perhaps a fulcrum of the cosmos? With the realization that the heart was just a really efficient pump, they heaved an unimpressed sigh and started thinking of how the mind might be the center of the universe.

From then on, we began to claim the mind as the major focal point to our studies. We began to look at the ideas of the ancients as superstitious beliefs, irrelevant in a world now ruled by the scientific method.

That is until HeartMath came onboard.[1]

The concept started before them, but we've seen some pretty amazing studies coming from the Institute of HeartMath (and others) that suggest the heart has such a bigger story than merely being a blood-pumping machine.

We've discovered that the heart has a brain—its own independent nervous system with at least 40,000 neurons (nerve cells) functioning within it. The heart's brain relays information back and forth between it and the brain within our head. We've found that the heart sends more information upward than the brain sends downward.

Think about heart transplantation. Through the miracle of modern medicine, we have found a way to bypass the heart, providing oxygen and circulation to the body while we remove a diseased heart and transplant it with a healthier one. When you do this, you have to disconnect the heart from its plumbing as well as its neurological connections, mainly associated with the nerves of the chest and spinal cord. These are direct links to the brain in our head. The challenge is that you can reconnect the blood vessels, but you can't reattach nerves. They can eventually reconnect, but it takes a long time, years at least, if ever. When you put a transplanted heart into a person's chest and reconnect the plumbing, the nerves don't come along with it. There's a separation between the heart and the head.

And the heart seems to do fine. The transplanted heart performs remarkably well, without much of any handicap. It can beat hard or fast, manage blood pressure needs, fluid balance, and fulfill all of its physical roles, even the ones we don't know much about.

Claire Sylvia was a dancer with an autoimmune condition that caused her heart to fail. She received the transplanted heart and lungs of an 18-year-old boy who died in a motorcycle accident. Claire got more than she bargained for after discovering that she craved beer and chicken nuggets—foods she had never liked before. After an extraordinary set of dreams, along with changes in her personality, she sought out the donor family and discovered that another person's essence—a soul and spirit—was inside her. She wrote about this remarkable discovery and how she learned to live with her new heart in a memoir called *A Change of Heart*.[2]

Ultimately, if the heart does not have to rely on the brain to tell it what to do, what does that mean about how it functions? It obviously can survive and act on its own. We know that the heartbeat arrives before complete brain development occurs. We can see and hear it on ultrasound between six and ten weeks. We know that the heart can survive and function adequately without needing a signal from the brain. What we are learning is the opposite of what I was taught in medical school; the heart tells the brain what to do, not the other way around.

As far as energy output goes, we have found the heart to be the strongest, most intense energy producer of all organs. It has an electrical field that is 40 to 60 times stronger than that of the brain. Moreover, the heart generates an electromagnetic field that not only permeates every cell in the body but also radiates outside of it and can be measured with present-day technology to about eight feet. The heart's electromagnetic field is approximately 5,000 times greater than what is generated by the brain, and there is evidence that this field not only communicates with the brain and the rest of the body but can also be detected by the people around us.

Might it be that when we get the heebie-jeebies around someone, or when we walk into a room and just feel something wrong without knowing why, or when we are around someone we care about and feel enveloped in a circle of love and affection, we may be tapping into something real and recognizable that is coming directly from the heart?

I think so.

We've discovered that the heart does not beat in regular metronomic patterns but rather in varying intervals, changing slightly in length from second to second. We first realized this when we found that children being born actually have better health outcomes the more variable their heart rate is. This heart-rate variability (HRV) is also related to cardiac health as well as to overall mortality; the more variable the heart rate, the better your heart health and your overall survivability or chance of not dying from any cause.

More important, the Institute of HeartMath has found that HRV can demonstrate a look or pattern that is different when we are functioning in an optimal emotional state as opposed to when we are reacting poorly to stress. Emotion seems to be the key here: negative emotions or just having too much mental chatter produces a random, chaotic, jerky pattern to the heart rate. However, when we are able to shift focus to the heart, breathing in a more rhythmic fashion and accessing a positive emotional state, our heart-rate pattern appears more ordered, fluid, and harmonic; it looks like a wave.

I teach guests at Miraval how to do this. They learn specific techniques to access this wave-like state, which HearthMath calls coherence, as a way to regularly follow their hearts when necessary, especially as a NET activity.

Isn't it interesting that a coherent HRV pattern looks like a wave—in and out, up and down, in a rhythmic fashion? If we look at the world around us, when we view harmony, we see this pattern. In his books, Dr. Weil talks about the breath of life around us. Everything is breathing: stars and universes breathe, expanding and contracting; a night is always followed by the day. Look at the pattern of the ocean on a calm summer evening. The waves calmly breathe in and out. Is it any wonder that the sounds of the ocean comfort us?

Isn't it fascinating that our own coherence may lock us into the same harmonic step with the breathing, dynamic world around us?

And from a spiritual perspective, is it any surprise that when we feel calm, fluid, and in sync with our environment, that we have access to so much more than when we're living in chaos? Is it a shock that this feeling of harmony makes us feel spiritually aligned?

Getting to the *heart* of the matter seems like it's the right thing to do. We should learn how to do it in a conscious fashion.

LISTEN TO THE WHISPER

Inspiration does not come with gongs blaring or fireworks blasting.

It comes in whispers.

Aha's don't typically slap you across the face; they tickle your cheek. They often come when you are least prepared—in the shower, on a hike, or waking up at three o'clock in the morning. They come in still, silent moments when your mind is free and open.

This is what the prophet Elijah discovered when he did not find God in the great and powerful wind or the earthquake or the fire but rather in the still, silent voice of a whisper.[1]

There is wisdom in this from scriptural traditions, but it also just seems like common sense.

Why would a *"Eureka!"* moment find its way into a fast-paced day full of frenzy, confusion, and chaos? It would be too hard to hear with all that noise.

Our world is filled with it; there's no escaping the clatter. It's everywhere.

We are charged with meeting this challenge. We need to fight for this quiet time, however it presents itself. Finding a space that is still, even, and slow is imperative to our health.

I do this with my breathwalking, prayer, and writing. Others find it in meditation, long rides, hikes, or swims. Art, music, and all things creative are moments when the muse is invited in. The shower works too.

Knowing that the whisper may not be heard during these times does not excuse us from offering the invitation.

The whisper is shy.

Any chance we can get to hear it we should take. Most of us could use the training needed to hear that voice and know what to do when the words come.

They are divine.

BELIEVE IN MAGIC

I am fascinated by four-leaf clovers.

I have one framed in my office. It reminds me to believe in the magic of things I cannot see.

The idea that they are real but somehow otherworldly is mystifying to me. Dr. Weil has written about his expertise at finding four-leaf clovers. He talks about hunting for them as a way to believe in this world of mystery and magic. He explains that belief is a skill to be learned, and such belief is a classic example of spontaneous healing—an aspect of ourselves that is lucky, mysterious, and sometimes elusive.

In his book *Spontaneous Healing*[1] he writes:

> Belief also strongly influences perception, determining what we
> see and what we do not see as we move through the world . . . with

that belief, there is a chance of finding [a four-leaf clover]; without it there is none.

Magic is hard to spot when we don't believe it exists.

During my fellowship training in integrative medicine, I had the good fortune to travel with Dr. Weil on a ten-day trip to Ireland. One fall morning, we were walking the grounds of Dublin Castle looking at old trees when I thought, *What a perfect time to find a four-leaf clover.*

Since Andy was the guru of four-leaf-clover finding, I called him out on the task. Now was an ideal time to learn from the master. He agreed to this test of worthiness, and we immediately started to walk around a patch of trees looking for a healthy spot of clover. I remember him peering down, looking around, not in any particular order or fashion, almost as if he wasn't looking at all. He seemed to not be focusing on the clover but on something else.

And then he abruptly said, "Nope, let's move on."

We found another clover patch. He went his way and I went mine as I looked on my own, eager to outshine my mentor. Nothing doing; I failed miserably. We started talking about him leading seminars where he would take people out on a patch of clover-filled lawn, teach them how to look, and then within 20 minutes, everyone would find them—sometimes even five- and six-leafed clovers. Amazing.

And then he did it; he stooped down and picked one up and mystified me even more. He gave it to me with a soft smile and a "Here you go, Grasshopper" kind of wink.

To this day, I have that clover in a photo album of that trip.

I did not find my own four-leaf clover until several years later, when I was practicing integrative medicine as a physician in Indiana. It was during a turbulent time in my life. I was beginning to question my spirituality in several ways, wondering if something bigger out there even existed. I remember one Sunday morning becoming overwhelmed and chaotic after going to a religious service—just feeling conflicted, as if I were cracking in two. I went for a walk in an apple orchard behind my house, and I was so frustrated I thought I would burst.

I remember asking a question like, "If you are out there, God, if you exist, then show me something."

And that's when I started looking down into a patch of clover.

I did this for five or ten minutes until I started getting irritated. What should I expect? I hadn't found a four-leaf clover after years of looking. Why would I find one now?

I started to cry, completely discouraged.

As I continued to walk, I heard a very still, silent voice in my head say, *Look down.* And in that moment, I believed . . . and there it was. My hand went right to a four-leaf clover. It dropped me to the ground.

Magical thinking. Faith. Spirituality. Healing.

It's all there, just like a four-leaf clover. You just have to believe.

And so with this belief, I know that healing is possible. I just have to look for it—hold a picture of it in my head, believe it to be out there, and go on a search to find it and bring it home.

So can you.

GIVE THE DAY
TO GOD

There, I've said it. I've declared my spirituality. Yes, I do believe in a higher power—the presence of something bigger than who I am.

You just read about the story that helped me safeguard that reality—to hold it close to my heart. I have a four-leaf clover to thank for that.

What I have learned is that if I start my day without giving it purpose, I usually screw it up. But when I dedicate the day in service to something greater than myself, it inevitably turns out better.

Not perfect—but better.

I have a simple, specific ritual that I do every day. I say a version of the Lord's Prayer[1]—the Our Father—spoken line by line, and done slowly with specific gestures from Jewish mystery teachings, known as Kabbalah.

This takes about 15 seconds, and after I am done, I usually find myself feeling more complete and fulfilled. Doing this practice makes me smile with contentment.

I feel it makes perfect sense to go outside myself and ask for guidance, inspiration, and direction. Opening up to something bigger than me, connecting to it, and then petitioning for assistance to be my very best is a habit that has served me greatly.

At the end of the day, as I look back, everything is better when I give it purpose and ask for guidance. When it's just for me, when I'm on my own, it's not as good. Inspiration serves me.

The whole idea of inspiration has a lot to do with breathing into ourselves the part of creation that is greater than us. In my heart, I feel breath is intimately linked to spirit. They are one and the same.

I'll talk about breathing in more detail as I offer recommendations for managing stress and improving emotional health. But I first want to introduce the concept of breathing from a spiritual point of view.

The word for breath and spirit is the same in several languages and traditions outside of ours: *spiritus* in Latin, *pneuma* in Greek, *prana* in Sanskrit, and *ruach* in Hebrew. Words like *conspire* and *inspiration* come from this root. To be inspired means to have the spirit within.

Interesting.

Rob Bell, a biblical scholar whose books I've read, offers a unique perspective that resonates with me and my spiritual walk. He notes that certain sacred texts from the Hebrew tradition say that when God takes away the ruach, the breath of life, we die and turn into dust, yet when God sends forth the ruach or spirit, we are created and life begins.[2]

What happens when a baby is first born? Is that first cry the shout of spirit celebrating a new life? What about when a man or woman takes his or her last breath? Does spirit no longer have a vessel through which it can dwell?

One of the many words for God in the Hebrew tradition is *Yahweh* or *Yahveh.* It is found in the Bible when Moses is speaking to God and asks, "What is your name?"

God says to Moses, "I am who I am" (Ex. 3:14). The Hebrew word for Lord sounds like and is derived from this same word "I am," known as Yahweh.

This name appears in the Bible over 6,000 times.

It was written in the Hebrew language, which has no vowels, so the written word for Yahweh or Yahveh was essentially four letters: either Y-H-W-H or Y-H-V-H.

In Hebrew, the letters are pronounced: "Yod-Heh-Vav-Heh."

This is known as the tetragrammaton and is where the word Jehovah comes from, even though that is an incorrect translation. In some circles, this name is never pronounced because it's considered to be too sacred, mysterious, and holy. The ancient Hebrews recognized that there could be no name that could symbolize the transcendent, unknowable aspect of God or being-ness. They never spoke this name except for once a year at a sacred time in a sacred place.

Rob Bell points out that ancient rabbis believed these letters functioned as their own vowels in the Hebrew language. They believed that these letters actually were represented by the sound of breathing. If they were the sound of breath, they need not be spoken; they were a natural act, not an act of verbalization. Therefore, why would you need to speak these letters when your being naturally used them as breath?

Could the name of God actually be the sound of a deep, full breath?

The Hebrew Bible starts off with God creating the universe and forming man from the dust of the ground and then "breathing into his nostrils the breath of life, and man became a living being" (Gen. 2:7).

Could this divine spark be in all human beings, regardless of whether they believe it? Could the doorway to spirit and a life *with* that universal beingness be only as far away as a simple, full breath?

Could we utter the name of God and tap into something sacred, mysterious, and holy? And when we forget to say the name of God, can the way we breathe close that door?

If the divine breath has the potential to flow through me, just as it could be flowing through every single person around me, might I want to know how to optimize it? Could it be as simple as "Yod-Heh-Vav-Heh"?

I find it fascinating and remarkable that the four-in-four-out breathing technique I teach in HeartMath—a 30-year-old biofeedback tool—is the same as a 5,000-year-old Kundalini yoga technique in breathwalking (Sa-Ta-Na-Ma), which is also the same as a similarly ancient teaching about the name of God.

Might it be, whether we think so or not, that this being-ness is in all of us? If we speak its name, might it continue to dwell in us as we consciously live and move and breathe?

By breathing the words "I am," I might fall into the present and forget what's gone on before or what might be tomorrow. And in the awareness of the here and now, I might find myself being fully alive and living deeply through the simple act of inspiration—allowing the doorway to spirit to open as opposed to slamming shut.

I choose to have the door open.

GET INTO NATURE

"My father considered a walk among the mountains as the equivalent of churchgoing."[1] Aldous Huxley, the famous author of *Brave New World,* said these words. His quote is telling about my own story of spirituality.

I was born and raised Catholic, went to Catholic grade school and high school, and for a time considered the priesthood as a potential career. I left the church in my early 20s for rebellious reasons, along with deep-seated questions about guilt and dogma and organized belief in God. I came back to my faith in a roundabout fashion.

I rediscovered my connection with a Higher Power ten years later through long walks alone surrounded by the beauty of the Sonoran Desert. During my integrative medicine fellowship in Tucson, Arizona, I studied Native American medicine and spirituality as part of my curriculum. I particularly resonated with the medicine of the Lakota nation and studied with an expert on indigenous peoples and their sacred ceremonies.

He taught me how to sing.

For the first time in a long time, singing traditional native songs, I remembered feeling at one with something bigger than me, a presence—an energy—that was larger than my physical self but that I was somehow connected to. Learning the songs and singing them woke something up in me that I did not expect. It was as if I remembered them. They came easily and effortlessly—and the voice that came from my mouth did not seem to be my own. Waking up to that presence was joyfully fulfilling. It was like being reborn.

That rebirth started with my walks. I found that I could pray outside—that God didn't reside in a building but rather was all around me. In the midst of quiet and the sounds of nature, I could sense a connection with the harmony of things.

Walking every day—even if it was just for five or ten minutes—by myself in nature allowed me to reconnect with what I believed to be my Creator. It became a deep part of my spirituality that I continue to practice today.

So if that's how you find a connection to something bigger than yourself, I recommend that you embrace this form of deep spirituality. Go for long walks, hike in the mountains, fly-fish, ride a bike or motorcycle, or do a trail run. Feel the pulse of the world around you.

It will not disappoint.

And if you can't get out into nature, why not bring it to you?

Hippocrates told us to revere the healing power of nature.

There is such beauty within the world around us—so much to experience and appreciate.

But all too often, we miss it, distracted by the pace of our lives, getting from point A to point B, checking off our to-do lists, or being preoccupied with what's gone on before, while mentally replaying it over and over again.

It is vital to bring the beauty of our natural world into our homes and living spaces. Nature keeps us mindful by capturing our senses. Whether it's the fragrance of flowers in your backyard, the wholeness and freshness of tasting vegetables grown from your garden, the song of sparrows and the buzz of a hummingbird's wings, the flow of water and explosions of color as Japanese koi frolic in their pond—all of these bring the now of the waking world into our lives.

We need this. Anything that helps keep us in *now* time and mindful of the space we live within is a priority. More important, we feel better when we are surrounded by the beauty of nature. A recent study from Harvard Medical School validated this. Known as the Home Ecology of Flowers study conducted by Nancy Etcoff, Ph.D., the presence of fresh-cut flowers in the home led to people feeling more compassion toward others and having less worry, anxiety, and feelings of depression.[2] Interestingly enough, having flowers at home helped people to feel happier, more energetic, and enthusiastic in their places of work. Bringing nature to us lifts our spirits with minimal effort and maximum reward.

Keep fresh flowers and other plants in your living space. Make a small garden, even if it's simply growing tomatoes. Design a water feature in your backyard. Put bird feeders on your trees.

Notice what happens when you bring the natural beauty of the world closer to you.

GIVE TO LIVE

The secret of living is giving.

I didn't understand the power of this simple act until I started doing it more often. I'd get glimpses of its magic whenever I found myself volunteering or doing something nice for others. With time, it became clear to me that I should make a habit of doing this simply because it made me healthier.

Let me explain.

My regular giving started in response to a talk I heard years ago about tithing. Tithing is a biblical practice found primarily in the Old Testament that has been taught for centuries in Judeo-Christian traditions. Conceptually it refers to making an offering of one's earnings (usually at least 10 percent) and giving this portion back to God in a spiritual fashion because it already "belongs to the Lord, and is holy to the Lord" (Lev. 27:30). The reasoning for this, according to these traditions, stems from the idea that our Creator has given us life and the capacity to earn; part of how we honor that gift is to offer something back in return. However, the notion of tithing has not been exclusive to Hebrew or Christian traditions.[1] In ancient Greece, the first agricultural produce from the harvest was offered as *first fruits* to the temple or church as a primary source of income for the maintenance of religious leaders and the temple facility. And in Rome, this offering was made in the household during daily meals as well as on special religious holidays.

More often than not, this form of tithing is still directed toward a church or religious institution. My wife, Sara, and I discovered that the same benefits of giving to a spiritual community could also be channeled in other ways—giving to specific worthwhile endeavors outside of our church but with a similar focus and intention. In each situation, giving in this fashion produced similar results.

When we first began tithing, Sara and I didn't have much money to give. I thought it was a stretch to give away 10 percent of my earnings every week, especially when times were lean. But doing this taught me several important lessons about giving that have kept me doing it ever since.

One profound revelation was that when I lived on a little less money or gave a small amount of my time, it didn't have a negative impact on my life or world as compared to what I had done before. What it did seem to make was a positive impact on whomever or whatever I was helping.

In addition, it also seemed that I got more back than I gave away. I know that sounds weird, but what should have been a drain to my funds almost seemed to work out like an investment—something I didn't anticipate. It was as if extra money that I didn't plan on having somehow came to me without me trying to get it: I would win something, not have to pay a bill, or get an unexpected gift from someone else. The resources I gave away seemed to come back in some fashion even though I didn't look for them or give them much conscious effort.

Regarding the giving away of time, what could have been yet another thing to do somehow would provide me with inspiration, energy, and passion. Unforeseen to me, I would find myself being able to do more or be more effective with my time. My schedule would free up due to a cancellation, for example, and all of a sudden, the time I thought I didn't have would appear. I actually got time back.

It was as if giving opened a doorway to receiving without me ever knowing where it was or how it got there.

But more important, the act of giving made me feel so much better.

The trick was taking the leap of faith that everything would be all right without clinging to an expectation or thought of an outcome. I had to hope that things would work out the way they were supposed to, knowing that I was on the giving end and that it was the right thing to do.

What I ultimately discovered was that I was living in a world of abundance, not scarcity and lack. Life wasn't about either/or; instead it was about both/and. Giving actually created *more* abundance in my life, as well as deep, profound happiness. It felt good—really good—to give; everyone could win, and I could feel deeply fulfilled in the process.

But if I ever found myself giving for the sake of getting something in return, it wouldn't happen. It was that simple.

Part of the paradox of this kind of investment was that the gift of myself, my money, or my time had to be real and filled with truth; and I had to let go of any idea of getting something back. More to the point, any time I gave for the wrong reasons, it would just feel bad. I would be left with an emotion the opposite of what I felt when I gave correctly.

Once I let go of the selfishness, giving not only felt good, but it also became fun.

Whenever I gave something—whether it was my time (volunteering), possessions (clothes, household goods), or money—it gave me energy, made me smile, and filled me with contentment. It gave me a keen sense of satisfaction knowing that I was offering part of myself for something bigger from which others could benefit.

More often than not, I felt better when I could actively participate in the giving without putting a whole lot of attention on myself. If I could get lost in the moment and just enjoy the process without focusing on me, the experience could be amazing.

I remember during a low period in my life, I got inspired to take flowers and balloons to a nursing home and pass them around to patients and staff. No one knew who I was, but it didn't matter. It felt wonderful to make these men and women smile, even for a short time. It filled me with so much joy to see the effect of what simple gifts of love and affection could do to people who might have been feeling isolated or abandoned. Even the staff was surprised and laughing. It made my day just as wonderful (maybe more) as what their experience appeared to be.

This happened several years ago. I can't remember what I did last week, but this memory is as vivid as if it happened yesterday.

Dr. Weil talks about giving as a way to feel whole and connected. It is, in his words, a way to be *secularly spiritual.* Giving doesn't have to involve a religious institution, although most spiritual traditions do applaud the idea of service as a way to dismantle ego. When we give, we get outside of ourselves and find that the self-centered aspects of our personality can be reshaped. As Dr. Weil observes with regard to giving in his recent book *Spontaneous Happiness:*

> Each day provides countless opportunities to practice putting others' interests ahead of our own to reduce the suffering or increase the happiness of others. The goal is not to acquire spiritual merit, increase our chances of going to heaven, or earn the admiration of the community. Instead, service is a way of acknowledging that we are all one and that the happiness of each is connected to the happiness of all. The more we can experience the interconnectedness of all beings, the healthier we will be.

This is secular spirituality.

Molly Stranahan lives with her husband, Tom Curtin, in the owner-occupied Villas of Miraval. An amazing woman, she is a former banker and business consultant who left the business world to study human behavior and obtain a doctorate in psychology from Rutgers. One of her passions is seeking to understand what drives people to do what they do and helping them make choices that lead to greater happiness in life.

We have a lot in common.

She leads workshops on emotional transformation and global change. She also speaks about socially responsible investing and the impact of financial wealth on people and families. She knows a bit about that since she is an heiress to the Champion Spark Plug fortune. She has been around money all her life and has seen much in the realm of what it can do to people's lives.

Molly's family taught her that those who are recipients of good fortune have a responsibility to help those who haven't been as fortunate. Molly understands the act of giving. She writes and lectures on the importance of generosity and philanthropy and how it impacts personal fulfillment.

I spoke with Molly about what giving means to her. In an effort to be more strategic about her philanthropic endeavors, and to determine if she could give more, she created a generosity strategy as a guide to follow whenever she considers offering a gift.

This is how she explains it:

My life is an experiment in giving and sharing the resources I have been blessed with in this lifetime. I use my time, energy, skills, knowledge, and money to support the increase of happiness in the world, particularly among those whose paths cross mine. I help people become more aware of the beliefs and values they are operating under so they can consciously choose ones that increase their happiness. I believe life is about change and growth and that we learn through reflection, experimentation, and the example of others. My giving includes kind actions, words of appreciation, sharing of knowledge, and gifts of time, attention, and caring, as well as money.

It is my intention to give joyfully, following my heart's knowledge of where my resources can make a meaningful difference to someone. I enjoy inventing ways for my gifts to create as much benefit (measured by my values) as possible. I try to be aware of opportunities to build more loving, supportive communities and to support the inner happiness of people I treasure. I want my giving to be an expression of who I am and what I care about in the world. I am consistently looking for opportunities to assist in enhancing the happiness and functioning of those I care about and want to respond in the moment they occur. I make my decisions by asking these questions:

- **Does this bring me joy?** Does it feel *right* and *good?* Is it based on love and caring? If I feel in any way that there is a "should" to the giving, then the answer is no until examination can change the "should" into a joyful desire.

- **Does this gift make a meaningful difference to the recipient?** How does this gift serve the individual's well-being? Is it empowering? What is truly needed? What is the message of this gift? What way might the most benefit be obtained from this gift?

- **Am I the right person to be doing this?** Is this uniquely mine to do?

I try to record my experiments and explorations in a generosity journal and regularly reflect on them and their impact (including on my life and finances). I am looking for ways to share the stories of my experiences to inspire others to consider new giving options for themselves and their families. Since this is an experiment in generosity, I consciously choose not to commit to a dollar amount to give or to focus on deadlines. My process is to be responsive to opportunities that call to me in the moment and to respond based on intuition and what my heart says just as much as what logic might dictate. My goal is to be responsible for the impact of my choices and action on others by constantly striving to be open and honest.[2]

Fundamentally, Molly continues to give because, in her words, "Generosity increases my happiness." Just as with any tool or strategy that is used to improve balance, continued giving restores health and harmony to the spirit.

Molly has figured it out. It works for me as well.

Give it a try.

And so with your spiritual toolbox in tow, the next step along the journey steers us toward emotional management. I define *emotion* as "energy in motion." This is why exercise is such a great strategy for dealing with stress. When you can move some of that energy around, it doesn't stay stuck. We can release it. When our feelings have no place to go, they stay trapped inside, looking for a way to come out. The body stores this as tension and tightness. Trigger points in muscles lurk in the places where unexpressed emotion resides. Impulsivity is also an option for this stuck energy to express itself, exploding out of us in behaviors that we know we shouldn't be doing when we're in the right frame of mind. And yet we do them, shaking our heads and wondering why.

Emotional health not only focuses on the feelings we might have; it also relates to how we express them in the company of others. Positive, nurturing relationships are a manifestation of healthy emotions. Negative emotional states break the bonds of friendship, loyalty, and trust, all of which impact how we relate to others in the world. Finding ways to deal with feelings effectively as they occur in the moment and beyond significantly impacts every relationship we have. This is what defines emotional intelligence: how we manage our state and how we relate to others. We should learn every trick in the book.

The next section gives you my best strategies for creating higher levels of emotional intelligence and health.

YOUR
EMOTIONAL
HEALTH
AND STRESS
MANAGEMENT

BREATHE

Breathing correctly is the master key to wellness. It provides the way through every door that blocks the feeling of health and vitality. On one hand, breathing can make you alert and activated and on the other, calm and relaxed . . . but only if you know how to get there.

Besides blinking your eyes, breathing is the only thing you can do both consciously and unconsciously. The breath speaks directly to the autonomic (or automatic) nervous system—that part of the body that functions without you having to think about it. There are two parts to this nervous system: alert or on and relaxed or off, with a continuum between. Breathing offers one of the signals that dictate how your nervous system will respond. Most of us are familiar with the on button but have no clue how to dial this response down or off.

I see so many guests who have issues with sleeping simply because they cannot turn off their minds. Their bodies are completely exhausted, and yet the thoughts in their head (I call this *monkey brain*) have hijacked their ability to become quiet and ease themselves into a state of calm. Medicine—either from the pharmaceutical industry or the health-food store—will not work in this case. Learning how to breathe will.

I was talking to a guest who smokes cigarettes because they relax her. How can ingesting a stimulant (in this case, nicotine) create a state of calm? In two ways: first it satisfies a dependent need for the chemical. But second and more important, it causes you to take a proper deep breath. Most people who smoke cigarettes rarely breathe shallowly while smoking. Rather, they take a deep in-breath, hold it for a time, and then breathe out deeply, often exhaling more than they inhale to get out all of the smoke. This is the perfect recipe for deep relaxation (without the cigarettes). I teach this technique to every guest I see. Smokers will take several seven-minute breaks to excuse themselves from the world and do these deep-breathing exercises; what a brilliant idea. I tell them to experiment doing the same thing without lighting up. After seven minutes, a feeling of relaxation will usually follow.

The key is first figuring out whether you're breathing correctly. If you are doing this, great. If not, you should spend all of your time to get this figured out.

As a rule, most people with anxiety, nervous tension, insomnia, stomach problems, high blood pressure, palpitations, elevated levels of stress, or a monkey constantly screeching in their head will have issues with proper breathing.

Whenever I teach guests about breathing, I have them close their eyes and put one hand on their chest and one on their belly while paying attention to their breath without trying to change it. I have people sit quietly for 30 seconds examining their breath, simply observing what's going on.

Try this yourself.

What do you notice? When I ask you to focus on your breathing without trying to make any adjustments, what happens?

The key to learning how to breathe correctly focuses on two skills: understanding how to use your belly, and subsequently your diaphragm, to optimize the breath; and learning how to consciously change the ratio of the inhale versus the exhale.

Proper breathing is divided into three parts: an inhale should first cause the abdomen to expand outward, which is then followed by the chest rising and then the collar bones and neck elevating. The exhale then brings neck and collar bones downward, while the chest falls as lungs deflate and the belly squeezes in. Most people have forgotten how to use their abdomen—I'm going to say belly—to expand on the inhale. They immediately go to the chest rising. Oftentimes they may do this in a way that is called paradoxical breathing, where instead of the belly going out first, it will actually suck in. This expands the lungs while instantaneously shrinking the space of our chest cavity. In one fell swoop, we have created a breath that is shallow and limited.

Do this for any length of time and you will become tired, short of breath, and even light-headed. You will also give your nervous system an instant message of stress and anxiety.

Most people do this all the time.

The only scenario where this may change is when a person sighs, yawns, exercises, or goes to sleep. In that situation, for a brief period of time, you may find yourself breathing correctly and momentarily feeling better.

To learn to breathe with your belly, try this: pooch your belly out and then suck it in. Repeat this three to four more times without doing anything with your breath. Then, with your belly pooched out, take a tiny in-breath, and then suck your belly in while exhaling. Breathe out all the way until it almost hurts as you maximally squeeze your rib (intercostal) muscles. Then take a breath in and notice your abdomen expanding. Your chest and neck will rise on their own once you use your belly. Try doing this for eight to ten breaths.

Once we have three-part breathing down, the next key is to figure out what messages we're giving our bodies as we inhale and exhale. When we learn how powerful the ratio of the in-breath versus the out-breath is, we can use it to our full advantage.

Try this experiment: breathe in slowly and deeply, and then exhale as fast as you can. Try four to six seconds on the inhale and only a couple of seconds on the exhale. You will notice a subtle increase in alertness and energy. Try reversing this to notice an opposite feeling. Breathe in as fast as you can for one to two seconds and then exhale slowly and deeply, using your abdominal muscles to comfortably squeeze out all of your air for as long as possible, trying to get to at least a count of eight. Breathing this way can often bring about a mild feeling of relaxation or calm.

The ratio of our breathing determines what part of our nervous system turns on; we are on alert, deeply relaxed, or somewhere in between. By consciously shifting the breath toward a state of calm or relaxation, we can deal with stress the moment it comes.

I teach two forms of breathwork: four-in-four-out and the four-seven-eight breath. You can learn more about the former by reading about breathwalking in the next section. The four-in-four-out pattern I call "the wave" is the form I use to become calm. I use four-seven-eight to get deeply relaxed and to help people slam on the emotional brakes when they are going too fast.

This breath is important for any stress-related condition, from insomnia to palpitations and acid reflux to panic attacks. I teach people this four-seven-eight breathing pattern every chance I get.

You first want to place the tip of your tongue on your upper palate just behind your front teeth. Keep it there as you do this exercise. It takes a bit of practice to exhale through your mouth around your tongue. Try pursing your lips slightly if this seems awkward.

Exhale completely through your mouth, making a whoosh sound.

Close your mouth and inhale quietly through your nose to a mental count of *four* (remember your tongue).

Hold your breath for a count of *seven.*

Exhale completely through your mouth, making a whoosh sound to a count of *eight.*

This is one breath. Now inhale again and repeat the cycle three more times for a total of four breaths.

Note that you always inhale quietly through your nose and exhale audibly through your mouth with a deep letting go, dropping your shoulders as you do. The absolute time you spend on each phase is not important, but the ratio is. If you have challenges suspending your breath for that long, speed up the exercise, but keep the ratio the same throughout all three phases of the breath. With practice you can slow it all down and get used to inhaling and exhaling more and more deeply.

While I recommend doing four-in-four-out any and all the time, I often tell guests to try four-seven-eight twice daily as a practice with no more than four to eight cycles at a time, transitioning to the wave afterward.

Earlier I mentioned that the word for breath and spirit is the same in many languages and cultures outside of our own. Why is that? Could there be some connection between breathing and spirituality? Could we open a doorway to this world by breathing a certain way but close it when we don't?

I believe so.

Start by learning how to breathe properly, and then practice these techniques in a regular fashion. Make breathwork a ritual. It is a wonderful way to deepen spirituality and balance your emotional state. If you can influence emotions the moment they occur simply by changing your breathing pattern, you now have a skill to immediately change how you feel. Think about how powerful that might be to improve your emotional intelligence and ultimately your health.

GO FOR A BREATHWALK

Every Wednesday morning I teach a class at Miraval called *Breathwalking for Wellness.* It is one of my favorite things to do.

Breathwalking has become a profound wellness strategy for me. I do it every day and consistently feel the benefits it provides. I like breathwalking because I have a hard time doing sitting meditation. It's just really difficult for me to close my door, sit, breathe, and go into "om land" for any length of time. I have three kids, and they all want a piece of me when I get home. If I close my bedroom door to meditate, I am constantly getting bombarded with: "Dad, what are you doing? Dad, let's go play outside! Dad, when are you gonna get up?!" This last statement is an assumption that I'm lying down or have fallen asleep while meditating, which is often correct. None of this is helpful.

More than that, my mind is just too all over the place for me to quiet it in that way. I am active by nature. I love the outdoors. For me, movement can often silence the chatter in my brain—as long as I don't think about my to-do list or my back history. That is usually my challenge when I go for a walk—having what I call monkey brain. Breathwalking helps me to silence the chatter in my head. When I'm done with a good walk, I feel energized but also relaxed. It is one of the few practices I know that allows me to experience an active level of calm.

Breathwalking originally comes from a Kundalini yoga technique written about by Yogi Bhajan, Ph.D., and Guruchan Singh Khalsa, Ph.D., in their book *Breathwalk*.[1] The goal of breathwalking is to make strong, purposeful strides and walk in rhythm. You want to move at a steady pace but do not want to be out of breath. The fundamental rhythm of breathing is four-in and four-out, so take four short, segmented breaths in, one after another, followed by four, short segmented breaths out in time to your steps as follows: in-in-in-in, out-out-out-out. The breaths in should typically be through the nose and the breaths out through the mouth (although I often find myself exhaling through my nose as I get calmer). I like to call this "stair" breathing in that you walk the steps "up" to each breath and "down" as you exhale. Periodically alternate this with a fluid four-in-four-out pattern that I call the "wave," where there is no start or stop to the breath but rather a fluid movement from inhale to exhale. Just flow the steps into each other into a smooth wave-like pattern.

Another technique to use while you are doing this is finger-tapping, which involves touching your thumb to a different fingertip for each breath/step. The technique begins by tapping your thumb to your index finger, then moving to each successive finger across to your pinky finger (on breaths in) and then either starting over again at the index finger or going backward, tapping your thumb to your little finger (so you tap your pinky twice) and then back to your index finger on breaths out. This is how I like to do it.

Try it for yourself. Finger-tapping is not essential for you to do to feel the positive effects of breathwalking, but it helps to keep rhythm with my fingers instead of counting inside my head.

Uttering a mantra can also work to short-circuit the self-talk that is usually active and ongoing in my mind. A mantra can be a sound, syllable, word, or phrase that is used to consciously create change or transformation. Mantras originated in India, and their use and type vary according to the school and philosophies in which they were taught. They are an essential part of the Hindu tradition and are a customary practice found in Buddhism, Sikhism, and Jainism. For my purposes, a mantra can be quite similar to an affirmation. Again, affirmations bring a present focus on something I want to keep clear in my consciousness and try to manifest by vocalizing the words, either out loud or in my head. When I speak either a mantra or an affirmation, I find that the chatter going on mentally is quieted and I'm not thinking about the past or the future, but staying in the present.

The first mantra I learned was a simple four-syllable chant using primal sounds from Kundalini yoga: Sa-Ta-Na-Ma. The mantra describes the Hindu circle of life. It can also be a metaphor for transformation, and the literal meaning of each syllable or primordial sound is Sa-birth, Ta-life, Na-death, and Ma-rebirth. When done with finger tapping, the Sa starts on the index finger and goes toward the pinky, ending with Ma. Finger tapping is also known in yoga circles as a mudra; it can be done alone or with a mantra.

I've learned other four-count mantras and will even say affirmations like *I love my life!* to the count of four breaths and four strides. Even when I don't love my life that much, this allows me to "fake it till I make it" and can certainly dislodge any garbage I have in my head that I'd rather not be dealing with, thank you very much.

Try this technique for two weeks, and see if it sticks.

WATCH YOUR FOCUS

Focus equals feeling. It determines our reality even if our focus isn't real.

Let me explain.

When I focus on something, I put my attention on it. If I were to tell you to put your focus on your right big toe, something interesting starts to happen. First, you begin to use your senses to direct your attention to that place. You may start wiggling your toe or feeling it in your shoe or sandal. You might visualize it or look down at it. You might say "toe" out loud or in your mind. It now becomes part of your conscious reality, yet it wasn't in your thoughts ten seconds ago.

So part of our focus includes our senses—sight, sound, smell, taste, movement, feeling—either externally in our sensory world or inside our imagination.

Another part of our focus includes the questions we ask. Let me offer another hypothetical situation to demonstrate how we do this.

Let's say that my wife is late arriving home from work. First of all, you need to know my wife. Sara is rarely late. If I care deeply for my wife (which I do, by the way), I start to ask questions when she hasn't arrived on time. *Why is she late? Could she be hurt? Did she stop for gas? Why didn't she call?*

With each question, my senses begin to start firing off reactions and sensations without conscious awareness; I am bombarded by feelings. Personally, I'm a very visual person, so I begin to start seeing movies in my head. Each movie is accompanied by an intense set of emotions. As I start asking questions about Sara's safety, images begin to pour into my mind's eye about what might be going on. Each movie I see in my imagination leads into another. As I start to guess what could be happening, feelings beginning to build into a crescendo as the movie progresses. Remember, it may not be occurring this way, but my imagination starts to create a reality as if it were. My focus becomes reality, at least for me in that moment, and the feelings follow.

What would happen if I didn't trust my wife or if I was angry with her? (By the way, neither are true.) What kind of questions would I be thinking about? *Where the heck is she? Who is she with? What the *@#! is going on?!*

Much different reactions occur if I'm concerned for her as opposed to thinking that something rotten might be going on. A whole host of different movies would be playing in my head followed by their corresponding feelings. This is focus. The emotional dynamic it can create is impressive, especially when what we are focusing on isn't real.

Two things usually come immediately with each question we ask: first, another deeper question, followed by an immediate feeling. The next question goes something like this: *What does this mean to me?* Or more simply, *Is this a threat?*

If I believe that this potential reality is going to harm me in some way, I will usually have an immediate stress response, followed by the ensuing feelings that come with it. This stress response corresponds to a typical pattern of *fight, flight,* or *freeze*—meaning I may get angry or irritated, I might want to run away or do something to avoid the situation, or I might get completely paralyzed with inactivity.

If I feel that there is no threat, the stress response usually doesn't come, I don't feel as bad, and I can begin to create a logical set of responses to proactively address the situation.

Threat or not, much of this occurs in our head. The problem is the situation is real in our imagination, even if it hasn't occurred in actuality. Regardless of whatever is truly going on, the stuff in our head is real for us and has a direct physical response. A cascade of over 1,400 biochemicals are released by the body as soon as it senses a stressful emotion, whether it's real or imagined.

The reality of the hypothetical situation involving my wife is that she is late. Any interpretation beyond that is exactly that—an interpretation. And yet we often let our focus run wild, which determines our reality for us, imaginary or not. If it's real in our heads, it's real in our bodies. Focus equals feeling, which equals our reality, or as the saying goes, "If you think you can or you think you can't, you're right."

My son Kyle had a fever of 105 degrees when he was two years old. It started off as mild viral symptoms with some abdominal pain and a low-grade temperature. A day later he was shaking uncontrollably, and my wife called me, telling me to rush to the emergency room.

When I got there, Kyle did not look good. He was limp in Sara's arms, interrupted by what we in the medical business call *rigors*— intense shivering and chills.

Definitely not good.

Fortunately, we discovered what was wrong. He had a urinary tract infection that had ascended into his kidneys and caused him to be moving toward acute sepsis. Thankfully, with the miracles of modern medicine, he received a dose of IV antibiotics, and within 30 minutes, he was sitting up eating a sandwich. I often joke with Miraval guests that even as an integrative physician, at that time, I didn't want Kyle taking echinacea or seeing a chiropractor. IV Rocephin did quite nicely, thank you.

The challenge about Kyle's situation is that most young boys don't get urinary tract infections without something else being wrong. We found out that Kyle suffered from an anatomical abnormality that caused him to have vesicoureteral reflux. When his bladder squeezed, rather than sending urine down, it went back up into his kidneys and settled into his bladder, where it was a receptacle for infection. There are five grades of severity of this disease; of course Kyle had grade V.

The initial treatment was to give him oral antibiotics daily with the hope that he would grow out of it; otherwise, he would need surgical correction. Ultimately, he did. Fortunately, in the hands of a good pediatric urologist, surgery is 90 percent corrective.

The good news is that he had the surgery, everything went well, and today Kyle is fine—a strapping young athlete who plays multiple sports and keeps us all on our toes.

The problem, and the point of this story, is that I have an overactive imagination. Sometimes I lose my focus.

Two weeks before the surgery, I remember driving home after work and stopping my car in the driveway, when I began to daydream. I started to focus on something, and my imagination began to take over. Basically I asked myself a stupid question: *What if?*

Being a doctor, I know all the things that potentially could go wrong in a surgical suite. My initial "what if" was minor—what if this small thing happens? My imagination made a nice little movie of that in my head, feelings included, but it didn't stop there. I went from that little mistake in the operating room to another and another and still more, seeing it all happen in my mind's eye. Before long, I saw a movie of me dressed all in black at a cemetery, holding a rose, and dropping it into my son's grave. To this day, when I see that image in my head, it makes me cry. I remember sobbing in the driveway as I recalled this imaginary event unfolding before my eyes until I finally came to my senses and screamed, "Stop it! What the hell are you doing?!"

Of course that scenario didn't happen, but it was real to me then, just as it was real to me (and maybe even you) a second ago.

Focus equals feeling.

This is one of the reasons I keep a constant vigil on my imagination. If I catch myself daydreaming, I try to pull myself back into the present as quickly as possible. Sure, positive daydreaming can be wonderful, but conjuring up negative thoughts and images and letting them take me for a ride is a surefire way to create chaos in my life.

To get back on track, I ask myself questions that are proactive instead of reactive: *How can I use this? Where's the lesson here? What's the next right thing to do?* Asking those kinds of questions changes my focus and puts my attention on things that *can* serve me. It is an important part of maintaining emotional balance.

I also change focus by using my senses: getting outside and seeing something beautiful, listening to pleasant music, smelling freshly cut flowers, petting my cat or dog.

Sometimes I'll just focus on my heart. I'll touch my chest and feel my heart beating. Placing my focus here makes me realize that I need to get out of my head and into the center of my heart—that place of intuitive knowing versus logical thinking. When I focus on my heart, I breathe differently—fuller, deeper, more evenly. This slows me down and leads me to answers that my head doesn't offer. Following my heart changes my focus out of a stress response and into a place that is calmer, quieter, and more serene.

It is a place of emotional health.

DESCRIBE, INVESTIGATE, AND EVALUATE

One October evening in 2011, I had the great fortune to work with members of the Tucson Symphony Orchestra (TSO) using music to help Miraval guests make sense out of chaos—a daunting task.

Music is a wonderful forum for experiential learning. When we listen to a musical piece, it immediately changes our focus and feeling. Our reality changes in an instant. We are forced to grapple with that reality the moment it manifests. When the music is enjoyable, we are transported to a world of wonder. But what happens if it takes us to a place we don't wish to be? What do we do then?

That was the task at hand for me and the members of the TSO Brass Quintet.

The musicians played a piece called "Quintet for Brass Instruments" to an eager audience that filled the auditorium. Our seminar's goal was to learn tools to cope with the difficult or confusing parts of life and react to the world with more grace. As a result, the music to be played was supposed to be a challenge to the ears. Somehow we were to find a way to reinterpret the chaos, but even with that expectation, the melody (if that's what you called it) was difficult to listen to.

In response to the performance, we received opening comments like, "I tried to like it, but just couldn't" and "It made me feel uncomfortable." Someone even said, "I considered leaving but decided not to."

To me, the piece felt like the soundtrack of a horror movie. It was marvelously played, amazingly complex, but all over the place—choppy and unpredictable. I couldn't get on top of it or find any kind of flow to the rhythms. It was challenging enough to hang on. I was thankful when the piece was over.

A colorful New Yorker in the crowd said, "It was just like being on the subway, and I came to Miraval to get away from all of that!"

Shawn Campbell is the director of education and community engagement for the TSO, and she's one of the reasons I got the chance to work with these amazing musicians. She and I were monitoring the crowd for comments.

Shawn taught a process called DIE, an acronym standing for a three-step method to analyze complex situations:

1. Describe

2. Investigate

3. Evaluate

The first step in the process is to *describe* the facts of the situation and the sensations that come with it. Naming the feeling can often interrupt the emotional ride it takes us on, especially when we do so without judgment. It gives us time to probe further into the situation, especially when we catch ourselves getting lost in reaction. In the case of "Quintet for Brass," the key starting place was naming exactly how the piece made us feel. This can help us begin to recognize the difference between the facts regarding the music and our personal feelings about it.

Once the description occurs with its various flavors, we can then proceed to step two: *investigate.* The alternative is letting our emotions take us away.

This regularly happens. More often than not, we react and go for a ride.

Proceeding to the investigation step makes use of a basic idea: oftentimes, we don't have all the answers. Acquiring more facts before responding can be critical in coming to the right conclusion about a particular situation.

Have you ever found yourself focusing on something you were confident to be true, only to find out that it was misinterpreted and your response was wrong based on what you came to discover?

We feel badly when we assume incorrectly. This happens all the time without much conscious thought—but it might not if we probe further beforehand.

We discovered that the cacophonous music we heard was written by Alvin Etler as an homage to his son, who fought and died in the Korean War. "Quintet for Brass Instruments" was a monument to his son dying before his time. Caught in a battle without glory or heroism in a place far away from his home and friends, a boy died and left his father shattered by grief, with only music to give him solace.

It was a father's single tribute.

What an amazing act to interpret war in its true guise, not as the "Battle Hymn of the Republic" but as chaos, confusion, turbulence, and turmoil.

And with that realization, everything changed.

Suddenly as the music was replayed, it became beautiful in its commotion, majestic in its unruliness. I could feel war and a father's despair as I found myself fighting through the mine fields of commotion and disarray. Suddenly it all made sense, whereas before it was total chaos; and that clarity completely changed my perspective.

It was a complete reversal.

How can the same music played only minutes apart make me feel entirely different with just a bit more awareness?

It makes me think of all the times I've jumped to conclusions, convinced that my judgment was true.

Maybe not.

And that takes us to step three: *evaluate.* Take the new information and piece it together from a different point of view to see if it may take on new meaning.

Maybe next time I'll separate the facts from the feelings; maybe I'll get curious and look for more pieces to the puzzle. Maybe I'll remember that thoughts are things—that focus equals feeling, but feeling may not be factual. The thoughts in my head, the lump in my throat, and the churning in my gut may not be right or even real, for that matter.

And maybe I'll free myself from judgment, find a new perspective, ask a fresh set of questions, evaluate what *really* is real, and expand my awareness. With that skill, might I see the world in a completely different light? If I can transform negative emotions into more constructive or proactive ones—in the heat of the moment when I need it the most—might that make significant improvements to my emotional health?

Maybe.

SWING AND
A PRAYER

One of the fabulous programs Miraval has to offer to guests is their challenge activities. You may have seen these on Oprah's or Ellen's television shows: scared individuals strapped to ropes and pulleys, screaming for their lives as they swing from poles, balance on tightropes, or climb 40-foot ladders.

My wife, Sara, had the opportunity to experience this while I was away with Kyle in Florida at a football tournament. She spent the weekend at Miraval with a group of ladies, including a dear friend of ours who had recently turned 50. They all participated in a challenge called Swing and a Prayer.

In the Miraval guidebook, the description of this particular activity reads something like this: "Face your doubt, insecurity, and fear as you swing from a 35-foot cable above the desert floor."

Sound like fun?

Just ask Oprah's friend Gayle King, who did it and has a healthy fear of heights. She said this about the experience: "That was very frightening to me, and I will never do it again."[1]

My wife and her friends wanted to try it. Basically, the challenge involves being attached to a cable and then getting hoisted up 35 feet in the air, where you stay until you make the choice to let go, after which you swing back and forth like the pendulum of a clock.

Swing and a Prayer actually requires a fair amount of teamwork, as the outdoor adventure guides who lead the activity give everyone jobs to perform: positioning a ladder for the climber to ascend, spotting for trouble as you go up the ladder, being attached to the cable by the guide, hauling the ladder away, and working together to hoist the person upward by pulling on a fairly thick rope in the opposite direction—sort of like a single-minded tug of war. Once the person is up in the air, it's his or her decision to let go and swing.

This is what I love about Miraval's challenges. They can be such a metaphor for change. All kinds of resistance can potentially bubble to the surface when you're 35 feet in the air dangling from a rope. Fear, doubt, uncertainty, embarrassment, excitement, inspiration, and a sense of belonging to a greater whole are all feelings people experience. It's typically not a place you would normally find yourself, but the feelings you get can certainly be familiar. How often do they come up on a regular basis? What emotional patterns do we find ourselves playing over and over again?

The question is, when you are 35 feet up in the air, at what point do you want to let go of those feelings and swing for terror, joy, or whatever else will come along?

The challenge (pun intended in this case) about dealing with resistance is that you can talk about it until you're blue in the face, but what do you do when you actually have to meet it head-on? Your response to any of Miraval's activities may not only be transformational, but they can also be a memory you hold on to for the rest of your life.

Anytime you want to access the memory of what you did on the challenge course—the specifics of how you moved your body, how you breathed, what you said out loud or inside your head, the choices you made in the midst of intense emotions—all you have to do is go back and relive it in your imagination.

And when you let go of that rope, remembering that feeling of joy and freedom can be something you carry forever. When you let yourself swing, it's kind of like going back to being a kid swinging in the backyard, kicking out into the air, seeing how high you could go, and laughing giddily without a care in the world—perfectly present in the here and now.

How often do we find ourselves doing that anymore?

Neil McLeod is the director of Miraval's Outdoor Adventure programs. He was there with my wife and her friends guiding their progress. Before they started, Neil told the group to switch up the order of things: if someone normally went first, she should go last; if someone normally waited until the end, she should muster up the courage to be first.

The ladies each described what they learned about the experience by saying one word to encapsulate how it made them feel. Sara said, "Scary!" while Heylie jokingly offered, "Nauseating!" She felt a bit motion sick with the back and forth of the swings. Celeste, the birthday girl, gave "Exhilarating!" as her response, and ultimately, Kim finished with, "Sweet Surrender!"

Kim is one of the ladies in Sara's posse who's had a particularly rough year. She describes her challenge encounter with these words:

> The 18 months leading up to our trip to Miraval were filled with life-altering events, which I admit had me picking up pieces of bitterness, unforgiveness, and unmanageable anger. I was carrying those nuggets around with me in a virtual backpack everywhere I went, unconsciously back then, but now in hindsight, it is so obvious.
>
> When I arrived at Miraval with three of my best girlfriends, we began signing up for classes, and the one chosen for our second morning was Swing and a Prayer. I read the description and understood the concept of the challenge as a moment of unpacking something internally, admitting the weight it carried in my life, praying, and then letting it go. I

took the challenge to heart and began to do some spiritual inventory, and slowly but surely, I began to realize it was time to release myself from captivity. The Bible tells us that we are not alone in our struggles. It was time to prayerfully surrender this weight that was beginning to crush me physically, spiritually, and emotionally.

I was number five in the lineup during the challenge, and whether I watched perfect strangers or my best friends I felt the emotional surge each time, wondering if I could truly let myself be free. The idea of letting go could be like leaving a security blanket. I had become comfortable in my discontent; could I really let go? It was too late to back down now! As our guide fastened my harness and handed me the rope 35 feet in the air, was I finally ready to relinquish what I brought to the top? With each hoist of the line higher up, I said another prayer. I found myself suspended with my feet dangling, looking out on snow-topped mountains, as I firmly held the black nylon rope. Now it was time; the virtual backpack needed to be lifted, and I felt it leave me as I let go, falling into exhilaration, freedom, and sweet surrender! Our guide walked me through the whole process, encouraging me to lay my head back as I swung. Never before have I felt so free! A Swing and a Prayer was exactly what this wounded spirit needed to move forward.[2]

Our experiences build memories. We want to be able to access the kinds of moments that reinforce our best emotions—those feelings that are empowering and make us feel strong, resilient, loving, passionate, adventurous, and courageous. This is the reservoir of memories we should rely on, not the constant bringing up of past failures, being less than what we are capable of. Accessing positive memories takes practice. It can be so easy to drum up the times when we didn't measure up, but challenges like the ones at Miraval offer us an opportunity to build our reservoir of moments when we did it right and anchor them to our lives.

I use words that I tie to a particular feeling. Whenever I say *daddy* it reminds me of hugging my children during their growing years, when they still thought I was a rock star and could do no wrong. I say the word during times when I need to feel warmth and love. I also love the word *yes*. I often say it when I need to feel capable in the midst of uncertainty. Saying yes repeatedly makes me feel like I can do anything that I set my mind to.

We want to find that emotional fortitude and resilience during the real challenges we face. Anything that can remind us to go there in the moments we need is what we are looking for. It is a most useful tool.

Remember, if you think (feel) you can or think (feel) you can't, you're right.

LAUGH OFTEN

I teach a stress management class at Miraval, where I spend a fair amount of time talking about the physiology of emotion. We do emotions just as much as we have them. A person with classical depression has a *look* to his or her condition just as much as a *feel.* These people appear a certain way—shoulders slumped, eyes downcast, movements retarded, breathing slow and shallow (if at all). This feeling translates into a state that they carry into reality. Laughter is the same way. Have you ever seen people laugh? What do they do with their bodies? How are their shoulders—forward or back? What about their faces and eyes—down or up? What about their breathing—full and deep or slow and shallow? Have you ever seen someone laugh so hard that he or she cried—crying with joy, not sadness? Have you ever been to a great comedy show? How do you feel afterward?

Laughter is good for you.

I remember doing a seminar with Dr. Weil on Cortes Island in British Columbia. He was describing a therapy called laughter yoga and wanted to try it with the students at the seminar. Laughter yoga is the creation of Dr. Madan Kataria,[1] a physician from Mumbai, India, who launched his first Laughter Club at a park in 1995 with a handful of willing participants. It has since become a worldwide practice, with more than 6,000 Social Laughter Clubs in about 60 countries. On his website, he describes laughter yoga as "combining unconditional laughter with yogic breathing." It is based on the premise that anyone can laugh for no reason. That is, you don't have to rely on humor, jokes, or a standup comic. As laughter is stimulated within a group dynamic, it begins to transform from a childlike playfulness into real, contagious hilarity. It is based on the scientific fact that the body cannot differentiate between fake and real laughter. The same goes for any emotion, so why not make it funny?

In our seminar, there were perhaps 30 to 40 people in the conference room—a beautiful setting with hardwood floors and bay windows displaying the grandeur of Douglas firs as the rain pitter-patted on the roof. We all laid down en masse, with Dr. Weil as the master-of-ceremonies. His job was to start us all laughing. He did it with a small chuckle—nothing big, really, just something light to get us moving along. The pranksters in the group began to chime in with seemingly forced bits of laughter, but it was funny enough to fuel the fires and get most of us to at least smile. It degenerated quickly into a towering inferno of laughter—guffaws, high-pitched squeals, low rumbles, and crying (I bet somebody peed).

The after-effects were amazing.

When we laugh, we feel completely different than how we feel when we are stressed. It makes sense to have this positive feeling more often in our lives. We need to laugh however we can, whether it's going to funny movies or comedy shows or spending time with funny people who put a smile on our face. We can even join a Laughter Yoga club.

It will serve us well.

FIND A
FRIEND
IN A PET

We recently adopted a kitten from the Humane Society. My daughter, Ava, walked through the aisles and claimed her first choice—an ebony female with whitish-gray fur beneath her neck and belly. She named her Oreo. There would be no more kittens to look at, and there would be no other names to give her.

We already have a dog named Cinnamon. We were at the Humane Society because my wife, Sara, wanted a cat to keep our home free of scorpions. She had heard about the amazing benefits of cats in reducing the scorpion population of Southern Arizona—especially the sector of land in and around our home. Whether cats are immune to scorpion venom (probably not) or are responsible for reducing the amount of little buggers in a dwelling remains to be seen. What we are discovering is that our precious kitty has given us so much more than merely carrying the moniker of Scorpion Queen.

"Oree-Kit" (my wife likes to nickname our pets) has provided us with hours of entertainment as she flaunts her friskiness in front of us and the dog. It is marvelous to see the utility of an old piece of paper or a fallen leaf in the paws of a pouncing kitten. We all laugh more as we clamor for the affection of this little marvel. She also likes to cuddle, so everyone takes turns holding her like a baby. We compete with each other trying to get her to purr, which feels delicious on the tummy. Oreo is all play in between moments of meditation, trips to the litter box, ingesting enormous quantities of food and water, or practicing her daily hygienic regimen (my kids need lessons).

The scratches on my hands and arms are too numerous to count. Oreo likes to play with Sara and me in bed during the early morning hours. Sara likes to sleep in, so this doesn't go over well. One day, before the sun came up, Oreo pounced on my head. It scares me to think what I must have looked like in her eyes!

All that laughter and joy, all those smiles and chuckles—they have to be good for your health, right? Fortunately, the studies confirm what we suspect to be true. Pets, especially four-month-old, self-entertaining kitties (barring allergies), are good for you.[1]

We've found that the positive self-esteem of children is enhanced by owning a pet of any kind. Cognitive development can be enhanced, as well as an increase in overall family happiness. Children who have a pet are more involved in sports, hobbies, clubs, and even chores; and having an animal in the house can help kids deal with difficult circumstances, like serious illness or even the death of a parent. Pets are shown to buffer the reaction to acute stress as well as reduce the perception of stress. They can increase social and verbal interactions across ages and timelines—working for both autistic children and seniors in nursing homes.[2]

I know several individuals who cannot tolerate cats for a variety of reasons—some immune-based, some not. If you are a dog person, go for it (see "Walk the Dog"). If not, what about birds, horses, or even snakes, lizards, or other reptiles?

Absolutely.

Pets fulfill the same support functions as humans for adults and children. Part of emotional health is having a stable community you can rely on, and there is nothing more reliable than an animal that wants love unconditionally.

It's a win-win for the giver and the receiver.

TURN ON SOME TUNES

The two things that can instantly change my focus are what I put in my mouth and the music I listen to. Whenever focus changes, feelings follow, and so anything that changes my focus can usually alter my emotional state in rapid fashion.

Food and drink are topics I will cover in depth because they can change your focus in a heartbeat and immediately induce a different feeling.

So can music.

We all have that one song—our song—that evokes an instant reaction the minute we hear it. Whether it conjures up feelings of passion or warmth, longing or love, energy or excitement, the melody or the words of our song immediately change our emotions, regardless of what we might have been feeling before.

Music has such a powerful effect on mind and body. Our bodies react instinctively to certain rhythms: we feel the beat, and it puts us into a certain state. Having been created *by us* to express emotion, music intimately speaks the language of the body. For instance, when we listen to slow, relaxing music, our hearts naturally beat more slowly, breathing deepens, and brain waves slow down. This is the relaxation response of our autonomic nervous system when it is activated. Music changes physiology.

Not only does music translate melody into feelings, it also transports us to memories we associate with those songs. Music can be a marvelous anchor instantly linking us to past events or situations and the feelings that come with them. Each song carries with it a series of remembrances and emotions that take us there the moment we hear the right harmony, rhythm, or rhyme.

Neil Peart is one of my favorite musicians and lyricists. He has been in a rock and roll band, RUSH, for nearly 40 years. Mr. Peart happens to be one of the best rock drummers to ever play the instrument. He remains feverishly passionate about the music he creates, the craft of drumming (as he calls it), and the lyrics he writes—all pursuits he has been doing most of his life. He also happens to be an accomplished travel writer, publishing several works of nonfiction about his journeys on the open road traveling via bike or motorcycle. He writes about the power of music being something that weaves together the soundtrack of one's life and times.

I completely agree with him. There are pieces of music—for all of us, I think—that incorporate the significant moments in our lives. They are our soundtracks. The minute we play them, they take us back. There are certain songs that instantly transport me to a moment I have lived several years in the past. I close my eyes, listen to these songs, and I'm there again, as if it were yesterday, all at the touch of a CD player or my iPod. The feelings flood back with the memories.

When my spirits are down, playing the right music can lift my mood and take me away from the funk I might be feeling. Music can also relax me, keep me calm, put me in a place of focused attention, get me energized, motivate me, or fire me up.

Hospitals use music therapeutically to soothe pain, counteract depression, boost mood, and promote movement. Music can aid in physical rehabilitation and induce a state of relaxation to deal with anxiety or bring about sleep. According to the American Music Therapy Association, music therapy can help lower blood pressure, improve cardiac output, enhance respiration, reduce heart rate, and relax muscle tension.[1] Moreover, recent studies have linked music with pain reduction and lowered anxiety in cancer patients, as well as improvement in the quality of their life and mood. Some research suggests that music can influence the production of neurotransmitters like dopamine and serotonin. These brain chemicals play a major role in mood, and when imbalanced, are linked to mental-emotional conditions including anxiety, depression, and addictive behavior.

A few years ago, Dr. Weil helped to create a number of CDs with music designed specifically to influence brain-wave activity, inducing a state of relaxation and encouraging the body's natural response for healing. I recommend these CDs to guests as a quick and easy health strategy to utilize within NET (No Extra Time).

Understanding the power of music can be such a powerful tool to help create the feelings you desire. I have a variety of music that can drive me toward the state I'm looking for.

Whether it's a Gregorian chant or "The Misty Mountain Hop," turn on some tunes and use music to move you to a place of emotional health.

Having gone to Emotional Intelligence University, the next stop on our way to wholeness, balance, and resilience is found in the material world, looking at physical health. We start with what to eat and drink. The challenge, right off the bat, is that nutrition has gotten overly complicated. The rules of the game have changed so many times that even the most educated of us have trouble navigating through these waters. Take bread, for instance: white or wheat? Do we look at calories, fat content, carbs, sodium, fiber, or high-fructose corn syrup? Do we even eat bread at all?

Help!

One of the problems in nutritional science lies in our biological diversity. We are all different; what one person can tolerate sends another to bed with indigestion. There is not a one-size-fits-all model for what we put in our mouths; however, there are some simple rules all of us can live by to make things less challenging.

In a world of more than **45,000** food items filling grocery stores the size of soccer stadiums (probably not that big yet), this next section provides strategies for you to live your life eating easier and better.

IMPLEMENTING SENSIBLE NUTRITION STRATEGIES

EAT RIGHT

When it comes to eating right, most people know what to do. The trick is getting it done. Following some of the other rules in this book can help motivate you to *do what you already know.*

Here are several things that can get you closer to the place of eating better:

Come to Miraval and sample the fare. You will discover that good food can look and taste great, that you can feel full eating less, and that mindful eating makes all the difference. You will feel satisfied, nourished, and grateful. If you can't come to Miraval, check out our cookbook.[1] It will guide you in the right direction.

Find a True Food Kitchen[2] near you, and eat there. This is Dr. Weil's restaurant concept. Having a meal there is an event you will not forget. There are True Food Kitchens in Arizona and California with plans to have restaurants in Denver, Dallas, Houston, and hopefully Boston and Chicago in the near future. While eating there, you will come to discover that healthy food is truly delicious. It's one thing for me or

Miraval's nutrition experts to teach you about the anti-inflammatory diet; it's another to learn by having an amazing dining experience. It's like an amusement park ride of culinary twists, turns, and loop-de-loops. Try the Tuscan kale salad. Yes, kale—raw, unadulterated, cruciferous kale—pure pleasure. Trust me.

Read Michael Pollan's Food Rules.[3] It is one of the inspirations for my book and is the only perspective you need to eat well in my eyes. This tiny paperback is a wealth of information on how to eat correctly. The first rule speaks volumes: *"Eat food, not too much, mostly plants."*

Enough said—really.

Knowing that I'm not getting away with leaving a section on food and nutrition this short, let's focus on some quick and easy tips to deal with in regard to what we put in our mouths on a regular basis. I want to put special attention on talking about the importance of eating in such a way as to consciously reduce inflammatory responses in the body. We call this concept the anti-inflammatory diet (see "The Anti-Inflammatory Diet" in the Appendix).

First, it's very important to note that this way of eating isn't really a diet. Diets are notorious for starting and then stopping because you can never do them for a prolonged period of time. Eating like this is a way of life. You don't ever need to get off of it, but more important, it's delicious enough that you would never want to.

Second, Dr. Weil has been one of the major innovators of this idea. He has written much about the anti-inflammatory diet in his recent books. His website—**www.drweil.com**—is a storehouse of information about the anti-inflammatory diet with recipes, an educational food pyramid, and information on how the diet may be applied in the treatment of chronic disease.[4]

We teach the principles of this eating style to guests at Miraval. Understanding that certain foods can either turn up inflammation or dial it down is an important concept to grasp, especially when medical science is confirming that much of chronic disease stems from out-of-control, under-the-surface inflammation in the body.

Inflammation is supposed to happen in response to injury or invasion. When we hurt ourselves, the inflammatory response creates a cascade of chemical messages and reactions to control the harm that has already been done, begin repairing damaged tissue, stop foreign invasion by infectious organisms, and restore and maintain body structure when it is compromised.

We understand inflammation when we see it overtly in action, usually after a physical injury. The classical inflammatory reactions are red, hot, swollen, and painful.

I won't go into depth about the pathophysiology of this response. Just know that our bodies do a great job of managing injury and repairing it. The challenge is that the response is supposed to first target a particular area, turn on at that location, and then turn off when we don't need it anymore.

What would happen if we couldn't shut off that response or if it went beyond its normal target? When inflammation goes on unchecked without turning off, we are in a constant state of repair. Have you ever hurt yourself or gotten sick with the flu? How did it make you feel?

Usually we are achy and tired. We want to rest or sleep. Anything we do fatigues us. We don't want to eat much in the realm of solid food, while craving fluids and things like soup. The thought of greasy, fried food turns our stomach. This is what happens when we are sick or hurt badly. Our immune system is spending its time repairing the damage and reducing the load of foreign invaders coursing through our bodies. This takes energy. It's the reason why we want to rest.

Have you ever felt this way without being sick or hurt? If so, chances are you have an inflammatory response going on beneath the surface, below the level of conscious awareness.

Inflammation starts from the fats we eat. We make hormones from these essential fats, some of which promote or dial up the inflammatory process while others dial it down. The problem stems from eating too many omega-6 fatty acids. I will talk about omega-3s in upcoming sections. These are the essential fatty acids that help turn down the inflammatory response. Omega-6s are the ones that dial it up, and processed food is loaded with these fats. This is one reason I want you to try to avoid foods in a box or a bag.

The ratio between omega-6 and omega-3 fatty acids in the diet used to be somewhere between 2 or 4:1—a relatively balanced ratio but skewed toward giving us the ability to turn on the inflammatory response when we needed to versus turning it off. Unfortunately, today's diet ratio of omega-6s and omega-3s is currently estimated to be between 25 and 40:1.[5] With that much inflammation going on unchecked and unable to be turned off, is it any wonder that we feel so bad?

We need to learn how to dial down this inflammatory response with food. The trick is to make nutritional recommendations simple enough to follow without having to think too much or too hard; that way these solutions become part of our lives.

The Mediterranean diet is a perfect example of a nutrition plan that reduces inflammation and lowers the risk of chronic diseases, while still being easy to follow, fun to do, and delicious to eat.[6] A recent study of over 1.5 million healthy adults showed that following the Mediterranean diet was associated with a reduced risk of overall mortality along with deaths from cardiovascular disease. It was also tied to a lowered incidence of cancer, as well as Parkinson's and Alzheimer's diseases, all of which have been related to overactive inflammation in the body.

The following suggestions piece together strategies on how to eat this way in easy, manageable steps. Eating an anti-inflammatory diet not only increases years of life but also improves life in those years; it makes perfect sense to have fun learning how to eat like the Cretans from Greece do.

USE OLIVE OIL ABUNDANTLY

The Italian word for abundance is *abbondanza.* It is often used in an exclamatory way to describe the richness, wealth, and fullness of life. This is how I want you to use olive oil—like the Tuscans do—with abbondanza.

Olive oil is a health food, pure and simple. The Mediterranean diet typically uses close to 40 percent of its calories as fat; most of this is in the form of good-quality olive oil, again used in abundant quantities. Ask a native Tuscan if she measures her olive oil, and she will laugh at you. They use it like water.

Good-quality olive oil is different from the stuff you might find at the local grocery store (although you can still find excellent versions at most supermarkets). First of all, you want an olive oil that is made in a delicate fashion by people who care about the process. The olive oil I like comes from the Tuscan hillsides south of Florence, where the olives are handpicked and then well pressed within 24 hours to preserve nutrients and flavor. Cold pressed, extra-virgin olive oil is what you are looking for, preferably organic and in smaller bottles as opposed to large vats or cans. The look of it should be a vibrant yellow-green as opposed to clear or pale-yellow.

Olive oil has the highest percentage of heart-healthy fats compared to any other available oil. Besides these monounsaturated fats, good-quality olive oil also contains large amounts of antioxidants, shown to improve cardiovascular health and protect against cancer. I include olive oil in my anti-inflammatory diet recommendations because good-quality products contain high levels of a substance called *oleocanthol.*

Chemically, oleocanthol looks and acts like ibuprofen—a nonsteroidal anti-inflammatory used for arthritis and other musculoskeletal pain.[1] The downside of taking too much of this drug is that it has the potential to cause stomach ulcers and kidney problems. This is true with most other drugs in this class. You don't have to worry about that with olive oil.

Connoisseurs check for oleocanthol by pouring a small amount of olive oil in a spoon or on the palm of their hand. They then slurp it up—this adds air to it, activating the substance like chopping an onion or crushing garlic. What you are looking for is a distinctive peppery taste in the back of your throat after about three to five seconds. Olive oil containing large amounts of oleocanthol will make you cough, it is so filled with spice.

That's what you're looking for in a good olive oil. Go on a scouting party and find a delicious one that will make you cough when you slurp it up.

Then act like a Tuscan, and with a big smile, say, "Abbondanza!"

EAT A
RAINBOW

I like to paint when I eat.

Whether it's the employees' daily lunch at Miraval or making food for family and friends, I love to create dishes that are pieces of art with lots of color. If it *looks* good, chances are it will *be* good tasting and good for you.

Dr. David Heber is the founding director of the UCLA Center for Human Nutrition and a leading expert on clinical nutrition, prevention, and obesity. His book *What Color Is Your Diet?* explains that most Americans live on beige- or white-colored foods—think chips and many snack foods, bread, pasta, rice, cakes, and other pastries. To add color to our diet, we must include fruits and vegetables that contain a vast array of phytochemicals. Phytochemicals not only give fruits and vegetables their vibrant color, but they also protect and sustain the health of the plant, protecting it from toxic chemicals, oxidation (rust), and even natural predators. We gain those same benefits when we eat these foods.

Unfortunately, most of us don't.

The average American eats roughly three servings of fruits and vegetables daily, when experts say we should be eating seven to eleven servings.

How do we change that?

Turn your plate into a coloring book. Make these foods your new art form and begin to draw. I like to put at least four to five different colors on my plate—the deeper the color, the better. Take the time to discover the different properties of these phytonutrients and their benefits, whether it's the cancer-protective effects of lycopene in red tomatoes and watermelon or the orange-yellow carotenoids in carrots and sweet potatoes that improve eye health.

You can also keep it simple and put a rainbow on your plate. Reduce your beige and white foods (except for onions, garlic, and cauliflower) and replace them with other colors—red, orange, yellow, green, blue, and purple. Plus, give your sweet tooth the satisfaction of the sugar found in fruit. I tell my kids it's God's candy.

DEVELOP A
TASTE FOR TEA

We live in a coffee culture.

All you have to do is go to the local Starbucks and you'll find that the world of coffee is bigger than Folgers or Maxwell House. The same goes for tea. We just don't notice it living in the United States, but it is easy to spot in London, Tokyo, Beijing, or Bombay—all of which are *tea* towns.

Tea culture not only has a long history and tradition, but it is also wildly popular today—just not as much in the States. Specialty oolong teas can cost thousands of dollars per pound. Same goes for some pu-erh teas, which I'll speak about later. Unfortunately, most of the tea we find in America is of poor quality, has a taste that is drab at best, and is available for most of us only at a local grocery store.

Develop a better taste for tea. I have been experiencing this world and its culture over the past ten years. Being used to drinking tea only as an iced beverage at restaurants, I never used to like the taste of hot tea. However, after trying a number of better-quality teas over the years, I've discovered that this culture is truly a rich one filled with variety, complexity, and nuance of flavor. Being Italian, if I drink coffee, I like it strong—mostly espresso. I began drinking tea in my early days of integrative medicine training, and for the most part, I've replaced much of the coffee I used to drink with tea—something I never thought I'd be able to do.

Tea calms me down more than coffee. It makes sense that this is the case when you look at the cultures of each. We drink coffee to get wired, stay up, and be focused. During afternoon tea, we sit back and relax, often enjoying the company and conversation of another. The ingredients of each beverage may give us a clue as to why this is happening.

First of all, brewed coffee has more caffeine than tea, about a third more at least. This alone can be more stimulating to the nervous system. All tea, including black, green, white, or oolong, comes from the *Camellia sinensis* plant. This is the only plant that makes L-theanine, an amino acid that produces a relaxed state of mental alertness, which may account for the differences between it and coffee. Several studies have found that L-theanine stimulates alpha brain waves, which are associated with this relaxed but alert mental state. You don't get wired as much if at all when you drink tea.

A number of studies show that tea has strong antioxidant activity, mainly due to its content of polyphenols, and this may translate to significant protection against heart disease and cancer.[1] Green tea, as compared to black tea, contains much more of a powerful antioxidant known as EGCG, which is why I like drinking it most. Research suggests that Epigallocatechin gallate (ECGC) acts as a potent inhibitor of inflammation as well as being anticarcinogenic; it kills cancers cells and prevents them from growing.[2] ECGC is found in high amounts in a form of Japanese green tea known as matcha.[3]

Dr. Weil introduced me to matcha over breakfast one morning during my first days as an integrative medicine fellow. I've been drinking it ever since. My first memories of matcha are still vivid. It was as if I was drinking essence of green; visions of springtime and freshly mown grass were overpowering as I drank out of an ornate Japanese bowl made of clay.

Matcha is grown in a special way: the most pristine tea plants are first covered prior to picking to concentrate colors and flavors, maximizing their antioxidant content. Once picked, the leaves are then stone-ground into a fine powder before being sealed into small tins. Matcha is made by first filtering the powdered leaves into a specialized bowl (not a cup). You then add hot (not boiling) water and whip the solution into a frothy liquid, using a specialized whisk made of bamboo. The making of matcha is an important part of traditional Japanese tea ceremony. People drink it because of the taste but also the ritual involved. I drink matcha most days for breakfast and sometimes in the late afternoon. I love the ritualistic preparation, whisking the tea with my *chasen,* and drinking from my tea bowl or *chawan.* It is calming but wakeful at the same time.

If you don't like green tea, there are other varieties to try. I like oolong tea but am especially fond of a form of tea known as pu-erh (pronounced "poo-air"). Its name comes from a town in the Yunnan Province of Southwestern China, from where it was first grown. Pu-erh has a strong, dark color and earthy taste, which comes from sun-drying green tea and then naturally aging the leaves in a process that causes them to ferment. The leaves are then packed into bricks or cakes. This has been done for centuries, and the process of fermentation changes the quality of the tea, along with its ingredients. A more recent process creates fermentation by piling, repeated dampening, and then turning of the tea leaves in a manner much like composting. Fermented tea is different than other teas. It has components similar to other fermented foods like kimchi, real sauerkraut, yogurt, and kefir. Healthy bacteria and other microbes exist in pu-erh not found in other teas. As a matter of fact, tea connoisseurs often suggest that pu-erh be put into its own classification away from white, green, oolong, and black teas. I often recommend pu-erh for coffee drinkers who are looking for something darker, bolder, and fuller tasting than green or oolong teas. Give it try.

You may turn away from being a java junkie.

MY FAVORITE BREAKFAST

I think skipping breakfast is the biggest mistake you can make.

At the same time, I know many people where eating something in the morning is the furthest thing from their mind. The thought of eating makes them feel sick to their stomach. Making time for breakfast while managing work, kids, the morning commute, and everything else that needs to be accomplished at the beginning of the day can seem like an impossible task.

More often than not, getting something on the fly seems like all we can handle.

Starting the day by eating nothing or with unhealthy choices is not only unwise, but it can often move the day in a direction that is hard to get away from. The minute I eat a typical breakfast loaded with carbs—something like oatmeal with raisins and a glass of milk, a donut or pastry with coffee, cereal with milk, or a banana and orange juice—I usually feel horrible. I feel wired and then crash energetically. I am not satisfied for very long and then have a huge craving for more carbohydrates. Once I start chasing quick-acting carbs, my day is a teeter-totter of ups and downs as my sugar spikes and then comes crashing down.

The good news about breakfast is that it can be very simple. I can usually eat the same one, two, or three things without getting overly bored with them. They just need to satisfy the requirements that keep me wanting to eat it: food that is quick, easy, and makes me feel good. I can enjoy diversity at dinnertime.

My favorite thing to eat for breakfast is either plain yogurt with a little whey protein powder mixed in or Greek yogurt (which has more protein). Having equal portions of protein with carbohydrate stabilizes my blood sugars and fills me up far more than eating something with tons of carbs. I get my carbohydrate from mixed frozen berries—organic blueberries, raspberries, and strawberries that I keep in the freezer and lightly thaw. I then add one or two tablespoons of ground flax seed as a fiber source that's loaded with vegetarian omega-3 fats and plant-based estrogens known as lignans to help protect against prostate cancer (and breast cancer for women).

With that I drink a cup of matcha green tea, loaded with antioxidants and certain phytochemicals called polyphenols for lowering cholesterol, boosting metabolism, and fighting cancer.

This breakfast is a great way to start the day. It can boost your metabolism for help with weight loss or if you are like me, weight maintenance.

Instead of a yogurt smoothie, I will often do eggs for breakfast—usually omega-3 fortified—and I will either buy egg whites on their own or separate them myself. I will typically use two to three egg whites with one whole egg sautéed or lightly fried in a pan with olive oil. To this I will usually add fresh basil and red pepper flakes and maybe some parmesan cheese. I will sometimes have sautéed spinach with olive oil, garlic, and lemon. This may take a bit more time, unless I do it in the microwave, which I may do if I'm in a hurry.

Eating small breakfasts with lower glycemic indices has been found to burn more fat[1] (up to 55 percent in a small study from Britain) than consuming foods that cause blood sugar to spike.

You can get all of these foods in most grocery stores, except for matcha. I often find the best matcha online, but you can usually find it in specialty or health-food stores. If you don't like matcha as a tea, try adding the powder to your yogurt concoction and make it into a sundae or smoothie.

LAY OFF THE PROCESSED STUFF

Of all the colors out there to eat, the one food color I suggest you downplay is white. Most white foods—other than vegetables like onions and cauliflower—have a high glycemic index, which means that when ingested, they turn quickly into blood sugar. This causes a compensatory spike in insulin, the hormone secreted by the pancreas that takes blood sugar and brings it inside the cells where it is used for energy. An insulin spike sends a message to the body saying it is under attack. As a result, the stress hormone cortisol along with a whole host of inflammatory mediators course through the body in an attempt to repair tissue damage and manage the threat of potential injury. Even if you're not hurt, this message is going on whenever sugar levels quickly increase.

Simply put, spikes in sugar equal spikes in insulin, which translates into inflammation and stress. Not good.

White bread—and other products made from white flour or white sugar (pasta, tortillas, cereals, crackers), white rice, white potatoes, or white fruits (bananas)—all have a high glycemic index (GI). This can be tolerated by lowering the glycemic load of a meal—by combining such foods with ones that have a lower glycemic index, like certain fruits (pancakes with blueberries, for instance) or with good-quality fat or protein, which will slow down digestion.[1]

But since we eat so many of these high GI foods and since they are ubiquitous in our diet culture, it is worthwhile to back off a bit if not avoid them entirely (at least until your free day).

One of the best ways to do this is to reduce the intake of processed foods. We live in a world filled with food-like substances that have very little life to them.

If it's in a box or a bag, it's processed, not whole. It's that simple. Limiting these foods is an important step toward health. It's a challenge to take all of these white foods out of our diets and limit breads, pasta, chips, crackers, and cookies. Think about making a proactive effort to eat more food that's whole or alive and less food that isn't. Limit fast, processed food to your day off if you have to, and eat more whole foods.

That's a great start.

PRACTICE
HARI HACHI BU

I first learned this concept from my friend and colleague Dr. Wendy Kohatsu when we taught together at Hollyhock, a retreat center in British Columbia.

Hari hachi bu is a teaching practiced today by traditional Okinowans (the indigenous people of the Ryukyu Islands in Japan). It instructs people to eat until they are 80 percent full. In English, the Japanese phrase translates to "Eat until you are eight parts out of ten full."[1]

This form of calorie restriction works because it takes about 20 minutes to feel fully satiated. Eating slower and more mindfully causes your brain to catch up with your body. Oftentimes, when we eat to complete fullness, we feel stuffed as our brains notify us to stop too

143

late. By stretching our stomachs, a vicious cycle of overeating is created as we try to fill in the extra space.

This is lessened when we practice *Hari hachi bu.*

When I talk to guests about this, I tell them to imagine their fullness on a scale of 1 to 10, where 1 is "I'm going to eat the house!" hungry and 10 is "Thanksgiving dinner" full. On a regular basis, you want to be somewhere between two and eight on that scale—never completely ravenous but not too full either.

Personally, I find that I have to eat somewhere between five and six times daily to apply this rule. My meals are smaller. When I do this, I have more energy and less mental fog, and I need much less caffeine. My blood-sugar levels seem sustained as opposed to being too high or too low. I am stimulated throughout the day, am rarely sluggish, and feel like I am fueling my body regularly in a nutritious fashion. The times when I do eat too much, I instantaneously notice a difference. I want to take a nap.

Hari hachi bu has been tremendously effective for me. As of the early 21st century, Okinawans in Japan seem to be the only surviving population that practices self-imposed calorie restriction. Living by hara hachi bu (and other healthy aging principles), almost 29 percent of Okinawans live to be 100—about four times the average in Western countries.

They must be doing something right.

"BATE, BATE CHOCOLATE"

"Bate, Bate Chocolate" is a traditional Latin-American folksong, often sung while mixing chocolate to drink at breakfast. It was first introduced to me by the children's cartoon *Dora the Explorer* one Saturday morning while watching Nickelodeon with my daughter. Now every time the Nicolai clan wants a piece of chocolate—usually for dessert after dinner—we sing this song and do the special dance. We sing/shout "Bate, bate chocolate!" and since the chocolate is mixed with a special tool called a *mulinillo,* the dance involves pretending to stir while singing.[1] It's quite funny.

So, whenever I want a piece of chocolate, I have to sing the song. That's the rule; my kids make me.

Good-quality dark chocolate is a health food. Eaten in moderation, it can often serve as a replacement for high-calorie desserts of poor nutritional value. Sometimes after dinner, I'm just looking for a taste. I don't need something huge—just a morsel.

Something wafer thin.

I typically recommend an ounce or two several times weekly. In all honesty, I'm all right with doing this every day. Obviously having great-quality chocolate around isn't a license to overindulge, and eating too much can certainly lead to weight gain. But I think it still is important to know about the beneficial effects that chocolate delivers.

Chocolate is a source of several different phytochemicals.[2] First of all, it contains similar polyphenols that are found in green tea and red wine. Research shows that these plant chemicals, especially bioflavonoids, may have a beneficial activity on platelets that can keep the blood resistant to clotting while also making blood vessels more flexible, thus reducing the danger of coronary artery disease. The fat that chocolate contains, stearic acid, seems to have a neutral effect on cholesterol, while other polyphenols may play a role in improving (good) HDL cholesterol while lowering (bad) LDL cholesterol. Another study found that 6 grams of good-quality dark chocolate (the size of a small square) had a slight lowering effect on both systolic and diastolic blood pressure.

Chocolate tastes delicious and stimulates endorphin production and serotonin, which increase sensations of pleasure, decrease depression, and control pain. Chocolate also contains mild stimulants like caffeine and theobromine, which seem to be implicated in reducing pregnancy-related increases in blood pressure. A study done at Yale showed that pregnant women who ate more than five servings of chocolate weekly reduced their risk of preeclampsia by close to 40 percent. Remember that dark chocolate contains higher levels of these health-containing antioxidants and theobromine as opposed to milk chocolate, which contains much less cocoa with far more sugar and saturated fat.

I typically recommend high-quality dark chocolate from countries like France and South America. You can also find good-quality dark chocolate bars at grocery stores for two to four dollars each. Look for brands that contain at least 70 percent cocoa. Higher percentages are a bit more bitter, so be careful when you go up. I often like dark chocolate with added almonds, hazelnuts, ginger, orange, spices, and even red pepper flakes.

Just remember to sing the song and do the dance before you sample.

DRINK MORE WATER

The earth is made up of 70 percent water, and interestingly enough, so are we. Every system in our body needs water to operate. Water detoxifies, transports, lubricates, and moistens, to name a few of its functions.

So how much water should we be drinking every day?

The short answer is probably *more* than you think.

Studies have been all over the place as far as recommendations for water drinking. In truth, water needs vary depending on our activity levels, age, weight, and exposure to different environments. Living in Tucson, Arizona, I have to drink much more water than when I lived in Indianapolis.

There are a couple of issues related to water drinking and health that need to be understood. First, low-level dehydration can produce a number of symptoms, including headaches, fatigue, irritability, joint pain, stiffness, immobility, and weakness in muscles.

It can also produce hunger.

Our bodies have a hard time distinguishing the difference between hunger and thirst. Oftentimes, we overeat when we are really in fact thirsty. The minute we get our fluid needs met, our hunger is satisfied.

Every day we lose water through breathing, sweating, and elimination (urine and bowel movements). We may also lose water as we drink fluids, like caffeine and alcohol that have a low-level diuretic effect and cause the kidneys to excrete more water. Foods and fluids with concentrated sugar can leach water out of our digestive tracts, causing us to have watery bowel movements. For proper health, we need to get a feel for how much water we're getting in our food and beverages.

Most of us have heard about getting 64 ounces of water daily.[1] This is the amount I typically recommend for those in their 50s and older who are of average weight and do moderate levels of exercise. If you do not fall in that category, I recommend that you drink more water. The Institute of Medicine recommends that men drink 13 cups of total beverages daily (104 ounces), whereas women drink nine cups (72 ounces).

For those people who exercise daily in moderate to strenuous amounts, I typically will suggest drinking one ounce of water per two pounds of body weight. At 170 pounds that translates to 85 ounces of water for me.

Whether you should add more water if you drink large amounts of alcohol or caffeine is a question that is still in debate. I would say yes, especially if you have any of the dehydration symptoms I mentioned earlier.

I would also recommend *eating* your water in the form of fruits, vegetables, beans, and cooked grains, which soak up moisture as they are cooked. All of these water-containing foods contribute to daily intake.

A quick and easy way to know if you're getting enough fluids is to check the color of your urine. If it is colorless or slightly yellow and relatively odorless (barring asparagus), you're usually good to go. Remember that taking supplemental B-vitamins may turn your urine a slight yellowish-green as the pigment from riboflavin (vitamin B2) spills out. However, dehydration is the most common cause of concentrated, deeply yellow urine that has a pungent odor to it.

The two tricks I've used to help me get in my water requirements are the morning pint and using water bottles. Every night before I go to bed, I fill up a pint glass (16 ounces) and put it on my nightstand. The goal is to drink this glass of water between the time that I go to bed and before I start my day. If it is completely full by the time I wake up, I drink it down. This gets 16 ounces in me immediately, even before I get going.

I also don't want to find myself urinating all night, which usually happens if I haven't drunk enough during the day and have to make up for it in the evening. I bring a calibrated stainless steel water bottle to work. It holds about 24 ounces, so I know I need to get at least two of those in during my eight-hour work day. I fill in the rest at home.

I like the taste of good-quality filtered water. It does not need to be cold for me to drink it, although I know some who prefer it to be chilled. If I want a different taste, I will brew herbal teas like Rooibos or Red Zinger. I also like sparkling water with a small amount of fruit juice—a great substitute for those soda drinkers who are addicted to the fizz, among other things. Lemon, lime, or orange wedges work as well. Drink up!

Knowing these simple food rules, our next step toward health looks to the realm of dietary supplements and herbs. As an integrative practitioner, I have seen this world up close—from touring facilities of supplement companies and organic farms to working with health-food-store clerks (some of whom are very bright individuals; others—not so much). This is a dizzying world, not unlike a maze. All you have to do is visit a natural grocery store and spend time in the rows of vitamins and supplements to see how confusing it can get.

We need navigation.

The next section streamlines a regimen of what vitamins, supplements, and herbs to take to optimize health. It does this without causing you to throw your hands up in disgust or frustration but rather to stay simple and focused. There will always be plenty of things to take. We want to have a practical routine that works long-term and enhances our well-being.

Simple is always better.

OPTIMIZING VITAMINS, SUPPLEMENTS, AND HERBS

OPTIMIZE YOUR VITAMIN D

There is a lot to say here, so I will try to rein myself in. If there was one thing you could do to optimize your health in the long-term, in my opinion it would be getting enough vitamin D. Making sure blood levels of vitamin D are optimized every day for the rest of your life is a surefire bet to prevent or better manage a whole host of diseases and conditions, including obesity, high blood pressure, diabetes, cardiovascular disease, back pain, muscle weakness, and arthritis, as well as upper respiratory infections, influenza, tuberculosis, MRSA, psoriasis, multiple sclerosis, and fibromyalgia, along with cancers of the breast, colon, prostate, and ovaries . . . to name a few. It can also help strengthen your bones, the health objective most of us think about when we mention vitamin D.

Vitamin D is actually not a vitamin but rather a hormone. The difference between the two is that the body cannot make vitamins. For instance, we have lost the ability to make vitamin C, so now we need to get it from our diet (vegetables, fruits, and their juices) and by taking dietary supplements. Hormones are made in the body. We can make vitamin D, and we do so by being exposed to the sun.

Our skin uses UVB radiation and transforms a cholesterol-derived precursor into previtamin D, which is then moved to the liver and turns into a vitamin D metabolite called 25 (OH)-vitamin D. This is then activated by the kidneys as well as cells in breast, prostate, colon, lung, brain, skin, and other tissues, where it does its job and then is deactivated.

The fascinating thing about vitamin D has been the discovery that every tissue in the body has receptors to bind its active form. Activated vitamin D targets over 2,000 genes in the body, and turns on the processes that affect over 6 percent of the entire human genome. That's a lot.

If vitamin D was only responsible for bone health, should it have this much activity elsewhere?

The answer to that is no, and to learn more about why vitamin D is so fantastic, you need to know the work of Dr. Michael Holick. For the past 30 years, he has been one of the leading experts on vitamin D research. He discovered the blood test we use to confirm adequate levels of vitamin D, and most of the recommendations I make about vitamin D supplementation come from his lectures and research articles (over 300 of them) and his most recent book, *The Vitamin D Solution*.[1]

Optimizing vitamin D is actually simpler than it seems. Here are three relatively easy steps you can take: get moderate sun exposure; understand about dietary sources of vitamin D, along with ensuring adequate intake of calcium; and finally, know how much supplemental vitamin D to take to reach optimum levels.

Regarding sun exposure, the time when we make the best amounts of vitamin D is typically the time when dermatologists tell us to stay out of the sun or put on sunscreen. Dr. Holick and I recommend moderate sun exposure. Here's how you do it: first, estimate how long it takes for your skin to get pink. This is known as the minimum erythema dose or 1 MED. Two to three times weekly, try spending a quarter to a half of that time exposing 25 percent of your body to the sun—typically your arms and legs. I usually recommend sunscreen on the face at all times to prevent premature aging there.

So, for instance, if it takes you 30 minutes to get pink when you're out on a hike in the Catalina Mountains of Tucson at 10 A.M. in late August, then spend two-to-three times a week being exposed to sun for 10 to 15 minutes before putting on a sunscreen of SPF30. I like to take walks throughout the day between seeing guests in my office. My walk usually lasts no more than 5 to 10 minutes, so I do this without putting on sunscreen. However, when I know I'm going to be watching my son's game for two to three hours in the Tucson heat, I'm sure to apply sunscreen to most of my exposed body, especially my face.

As far as supplementation goes, calcium and vitamin D play a vital role with each other. At present, I think most of us don't know about calcium supplementation relative to vitamin D. I can't tell you how many women with osteopenia or osteoporosis come to me asking for recommendations about strengthening their bones. Some don't know their vitamin D levels or have never had them checked, despite the fact that they are supplementing with 1,200 to 1,500 mg of calcium. When you are deficient in vitamin D, you can only absorb 10 to 15 percent of the calcium you ingest. Not good.

The first thing I suggest they do is have their blood level for 25 (OH) vitamin D checked. This is determined by how much sun you get, how many vitamin D–fortified foods you eat (there aren't many), and how much supplementation you take. I think an optimum score is between 40 to 60 ng/ml, where the normal range falls between 30 to 100 ng/ml.

I'd rather you get this test in the spring or fall and not in the summer, when your vitamin D levels will be at their maximum (although if they are low or borderline during this time, we know they will be low in the winter).

My recommendations for calcium typically fall in the category of 1,000 to 1,200 mg per day (the higher amounts for growing children into their teens and for women over 50). Remember, this includes the amount of calcium you get in your diet. Besides dairy products, other foods rich in calcium include collards and mustard greens, kale, bok choy, broccoli, canned salmon and sardines, fortified tofu, soy milk, fruit juice, and blackstrap molasses. If you supplement, I like calcium citrate best because it is more easily absorbed. Take no more than 500 to 700 mg a day, and take calcium supplements with meals. I don't recommend that men take calcium in supplemental form.

Vitamin D foods typically do not give you much; an eight-ounce glass of milk will offer only 100 IU. If you are unable to get out in the sun on a sensible basis or if you live in a place where there is little sun for long periods of time—anywhere north of San Diego or Atlanta— taking sensible amounts of supplemental vitamin D is a smart idea.

According to Dr. Holick and several other vitamin D experts, both children and adults need a minimum of 1,000 IU of vitamin D per day (preferably 2,000 IU per day) to maintain a normal blood level of 30 ng/ml or higher. The very conservative Institute of Medicine recently increased the safe upper limit of normal daily intake of vitamin D from 2,000 IU to 4,000 IU. This is not a limit, but merely an assurance of safety for such an amount taken on a daily basis.

I recommend 2,000 IU to most adults with the recommendation that they get their 25 (OH) vitamin D levels checked annually to make sure their levels stay in the optimum range of 40 to 60 ng/ml.

Simple enough.

TAKE A GOOD DAILY MULTIVITAMIN-MINERAL SUPPLEMENT

Unfortunately, I am not talking about One-a-Day or Centrum—sorry. My first complaint about such daily supplements is that they usually don't work. Most people rarely feel a difference from taking them.

One of the challenges of taking supplements is staying motivated to be on them for any length of time. My guess is that long-term compliance comes from noticing positive results. In the case of vita-mins and supplements, you should notice a difference. They *should* make you feel better.

I like to call this the *step up* or *step off.*

I've been taking the same supplemental regimen for several years now, so I don't notice the *step up* much. However, as I get new clients on dietary supplements, they often notice the *step up* as a subtle feel-ing of having more energy; they're not so tired when they start the day or don't have an overwhelming need for a 3 P.M. caffeine boost. Other individuals with high levels of stress may experience the *step up* as less irritability or a longer fuse; they don't blow up as often or as intensely as before.

The *step up* is a good thing. Your vitamin regimen should give it to you.

I notice the *step off* more often than the *step up* whenever I run out of my supplements or forget to take them (usually on vacations when I am trying to help my wife pack three kids into our van and I space out on my personal packing). Feeling tired or more fatigued as I catch myself yawning mid-afternoon is usually a sign that I'm off my vitamins. Deficiencies in vitamins and minerals have been reported in individuals with mood disorders;[1] correcting the problem can help in certain situations. Sometimes my wife will ask me if I've forgotten to take my supplements for stress management when my mood is off. Usually she is right. The reason why you experience this feeling is that the regimen is actually working.

Could this be placebo effect? Yes, but I have tried many differ-ent products over the past ten-plus years. Since I am in touch with my body, I can tell when something is working or not. I think most people can.

It's important to be wary of supplements that are very expensive, difficult to take, or both. But a solid multivitamin-mineral supplement is a good idea; it acts as insurance against gaps in the diet and helps compensate when we may not eat as well as we should or when the food we get is not as nutrient-rich as it should be.

My second complaint is that once we move to better-quality supplements, a couple of things happen. First, the cost always goes up—sometimes astronomically. Second, you often have to take things several times throughout the day. Companies that sell higher-end vitamins will argue that you don't eat once a day so you shouldn't get your supplements all at one time. I understand that, but I also know myself and I have a hard time taking anything twice daily; three times a day . . . forget it.

If I am trying to get people to take a dietary supplement or natural remedy regularly for the rest of their lives, the best chance I have is for them to do it in one or two shots.

Other things to consider are pill or capsule size, tolerability, and convenience. Does the product come in a packet, or do I have to count out pills and put them in a plastic container?

Ideally, your multivitamin should be a one-stop shop. It should give you what you're looking for without having to take a large number of pills. It needs to be convenient, portable, and easily tolerated. And it shouldn't cost an arm and a leg.

If you would like my specific recommendations, please see "Dietary Supplements" in the Appendix.

GET MORE OMEGA-3S

Snake-oil salesmen might have had it right.

Interestingly enough, the *actual* Chinese snake oil peddled by traveling salesmen in the 1800s came from sea snakes and was chock-full of omega-3 fatty acids.[1] Unfortunately, most of the stuff that was sold was probably fake, of poor quality, and horribly unregulated—not so far from our present-day supplement industry.

Traditionally, snake oil has been a folk remedy in Chinese medicine for hundreds of years, primarily used to treat joint pain. It was most likely introduced to America with the arrival of Chinese laborers building the Transcontinental Railroad in the 1860s. They probably offered it to their fellow workers to ease the bursitis and arthritis resulting from long hours of hard labor. Chinese sea-snake oil has been found to have more omega-3s than salmon, as reported in a 1989 article in the *Western Journal of Medicine.*

Similar levels of these fats are also found in krill oil—tiny, shrimp-like creatures found in icy cold waters and eaten in large amounts by whales. Other fish that contain omega-3s in high amounts are sardines, herring, mackerel, Albacore tuna, and Alaskan black cod.[2]

Omega-3 fatty acids are essential fats found mainly in these kinds of cold-water fish. Other dietary sources include grass-fed game as well as fortified eggs from chickens given a special feed that includes algae, alfalfa, or kelp.

Vegetarian sources include flax, hemp and pumpkin seeds, walnuts, and the vegetable weed purslane. The problem is that these sources do not give us the two types of omega-3s that our bodies best recognize and use. These are EPA (eicosapentaneoic acid) and DHA (docosahexaenoic acid).

For the past 30 years, we've discovered that in addition to treating arthritis, omega-3 fats can help prevent and manage any disorder that is influenced by an inflammatory response.[3] This includes heart disease, stroke, diabetes, obesity, asthma, and other lung diseases, along with several forms of cancer and autoimmune conditions like lupus and rheumatoid arthritis. Omega-3s are helpful in reducing cholesterol, blood pressure, and the risk for sudden death. They can also improve cognition and attention deficit, and help manage memory problems, depression, and bipolar disorder. The brain and heart have the highest concentration of omega-3s in their cell membranes, but all of our cells need them.

The development of any of these conditions may indicate a deficiency in omega-3s. So may the all-too-common problems of dry hair and skin.

I recommend trying to get cold-water fish in your diet at least twice a week, along with taking supplemental fish oil in capsule or liquid form. You should shoot for at least two grams a day of combined EPA and DHA. Look on the back of the bottle at the ingredients and make sure you do your math by adding up both of them.

Don't be fooled by the serving size or the amount that is specified under fish oil; it will typically be more than the total EPA and DHA and does not count.

Another problem is purity. Remember that fish oil comes from fish, which come from oceans, which are contaminated. You always want to look for molecularly distilled products certified free of heavy metals and other contaminants.

You also want to find a fish oil that doesn't burp up on you. There's nothing worse than having a fishy taste in your mouth throughout the day. Better-quality supplements will be "burp free" or flavored with natural extracts of lemon or strawberry. By its nature, krill oil does not have a fishy taste due to its different absorption. You can also try to refrigerate your fish oil to reduce the problem.

Because the average American diet is so lacking in omega-3s, and because they play such a major role in so many health conditions, I think it's vital that all of us incorporate more of these fats in our diet either through food, supplementation, or both.

THE MAGIC
OF TULSI

Let me share why I generally use medicinal plants over pharmaceutical drugs. Frankly, I think botanicals do a much better job with less toxicity than conventional drugs or surgery for the treatment of conditions that are mild to moderate in severity. Plants contain a wide array of chemical compounds working on a multitude of systems in the body. Their effects are not related to just one ingredient, even though one compound might trump the others in concentration or effects.

The coca leaf is not cocaine, for instance. Interestingly, the Andes Indians who use coca leaves do so to treat both diarrhea and constipation. How can this be? Coca leaves possess 14 bioactive alkaloids (of which one is cocaine); some stimulate the gut while others inhibit its activity. If you present the whole mixture to the body—as opposed to a single, highly purified version of one compound—the thought is that receptors in gut tissue can bind to the alkaloids that are needed and available to return it back to balance, disregarding ones that are unnecessary. This is a theory of how medicinal plants may offer more treatment options with fewer side effects because they are far more dilute and less absorbable than drugs.

Of all the medicinal plants I use, one of my favorites is known as holy basil. I was first introduced to this green leafy plant during my fellowship training at the University of Arizona's Center for Integrative Medicine. At the time, I was studying botanical remedies in Costa Rica with Dr. Weil, and I came across this fascinating adaptogen, popularly known as *tulsi,* being grown on an organic farm. Holy basil *(Ocimum sanctum)* is considered sacred in India. It is one of the prized botanicals used in the ancient traditional Indian medical system known as Ayurveda.

Through my research, I discovered that holy basil has antioxidant and anti-inflammatory properties, but what fascinated me more was its use by mystics and meditators as a *rasayana*—an herb to foster personal growth and enlightenment. Living tulsi plants are kept in many Indian homes, where it is believed to provide a sacred aura and endow divine protection to one's household; rosaries are made from its cut stems and used for prayer beads.

Holy basil has been shown to lower elevated levels of cortisol, the long-acting stress hormone produced by the adrenal glands.[1] High levels of cortisol can damage the cardiovascular system; retard immunity; create imbalances of other hormones; kill memory cells in the brain; worsen bone loss; increase carbohydrate cravings; raise blood pressure, cholesterol, and glucose; and accelerate the aging process.

Most of my clients have stress-related conditions that I am trying to help them manage. Holy basil is now at the top of my list of plant-based strategies to target such issues. My personal experience with it is that it lengthens my emotional fuse. My reactive fight-or-flight response to stress is much less intense when I take it. I find it gives me greater patience and more of an opportunity to be mindful.

I have been recommending holy basil for several years, and most of my clients swear by it. It is one of the few remedies I'd take with me if I were stranded on a deserted island.

I like holy basil for individuals whose elevated stress levels are causing health problems, and I use it as an alternative to prescription drugs for mild to moderate mood disorders.

I typically recommend extracts standardized to 2 percent ursolic acid in 400-milligram capsules at a dosage of two capsules one to two times daily with food. It also comes in the form of a non-caffeinated tea, known as tulsi. The tea has a subtle herbal aroma and taste that is not strong. I recommend one to two cups of this daily for starters.

LEARN MORE ABOUT 'SHROOMS

No, I'm not talking about *those* kind of mushrooms.

I'm referring to mushrooms that have medicinal properties outside of the consciousness-altering spectrum.

I love mushrooms. Unfortunately, the ones that we are most familiar with are probably not the best for us. I generally don't recommend eating white or button mushrooms usually found in supermarkets. The same applies for portobello and crimini mushrooms, which fall into a similar category. These are among a number of different foods—including things like celery, peanuts, and smoked foods or some pickled products—that contain natural carcinogens. Regardless of whether you decide to eat these, it's important to know that you should never eat mushrooms raw; cooking them over high heat will break down most of these toxins.

Every so often, I may eat a portobello mushroom or two, but I think it's a great idea to know about other mushrooms that do not contain some of these toxic compounds but rather have a whole host of health-promoting properties.

The edible mushrooms I recommend are shiitake, oyster mushrooms, maitake, enoki, and one known as the almond mushroom (*Agaricus brazilliensis*). Most of these edibles have significant anti-cancer and immune boosting effects.[1] The almond mushroom is sweet, with a pronounced almond-extract flavor. I had a pizza with these on it at True Food Kitchen; it was amazing—like eating Italian almond cookies.

Look for these and eat them any chance you get.

My favorite mushrooms to use as supplements are Cordyceps and Reishi.[2] Cordycep mushrooms have been used by Olympic athletes in China for decades.[3] Their use in traditional Chinese medicine (TCM) has been documented in ancient texts that date back to the 7th century. Cordyceps has been compared to Asian ginseng as a rare, adaptogenic herb of high esteem—adaptogens being nontoxic plants that help the body adapt to stress of all kinds, bringing it back into balance.[4] In the past, Cordyceps was taken by Chinese royalty, since they were the only ones who had access to it and could afford the cost. To this day, wild-crafted versions are pricey, going for as much as $400 for 40 grams.

The growth cycle of *Cordyceps sinensis* gets a bit gross. The Chinese name for this fungus is translated as "summer plant, winter worm." This is because Cordyceps grows as a parasite out of the heads of bugs, each species targeting a specific kind of insect. Any bug infected by the spores in wintertime will be dead by summer—hence the name. *Cordyceps sinensis* is known as the caterpillar fungus for obvious reasons. It grows out of larva from the Himalayan bat moth and was first found in the mountain regions of western China and Tibet several centuries ago. Herdsmen noticed that their animals were more energized and lively after feasting on large patches of mushroom-infested caterpillars. Fortunately (for our sake), modern technology has allowed for Cordyceps to be grown in large quantities under controlled environments, making it much more affordable . . . and without the bugs.

It is said that taking Cordyceps can enhance athletic performance, overcome general weakness and fatigue, improve sexual vigor, strengthen the immune system, promote mental energy, and act as a tonic for physical stamina and longevity. Recent research[5, 6] on Cordyceps has found it to be beneficial on liver and kidney disorders, elevated cholesterol, low libido, and fatigue. It also has anticancer effects, antioxidant activity, and immune-modulating effects, as well as studies suggesting that it can improve lung function and aerobic capacity.

Reishi (*Ganoderma lucidum*) has been used in TCM for over 2,000 years. It is known as *ling zhi* or the "mushroom of immortality" in China, while in Japan, it is referred to as *mannentake* or "the 10,000 year mushroom." Reishi grows on hardwoods like maple, oak, and elm trees, preferring tropical and subtropical climates. It is strictly used medicinally, being too woody, hard, and bitter for consumption. Like Cordyceps, it is very rare to find in the wild and is grown commercially under environmentally stable conditions. This makes reishi available to everyone at a tolerable expense as opposed to being relegated to the rich as the "medicine of kings."

Reishi is one of the great longevity tonics of Chinese medicine used to improve vitality, strength, and stamina. The Japanese government officially lists reishi mushrooms as a cancer treatment. Asian research has confirmed its use as an adjunctive treatment with chemotherapy as it enhances the immune response, alleviates nausea, protects kidney function, and helps safeguard damage to DNA by raising antioxidant activity.[7]

The active ingredients of reishi and other mushrooms that are so beneficial to health come from complex sugars known as polysaccharides occurring in their cell walls. Specific polysaccharides, called Beta-D-glucans, have been found to boost immune system activity. This is what makes mushrooms like reishi so popular in helping against diseases like AIDS and cancer. A National Cancer Institute study showed that injecting tumors with these polysaccharide derivatives could reduce their size as well as recruit more T-cell macrophages, resulting in accelerated cell death at the tumor site.[8] Beta-glucan supplements are widely promoted commercially for boosting immunity.

I'd rather recommend mushrooms.

Another important health component in reishi is its *triterpene* compounds. These are steroid-like molecules that have anti-inflammatory properties and inhibit histamine release.[9] This is one of the reasons why I use combinations of Cordyceps and reishi to help people with lung problems. They are used in several traditional Chinese formulas that treat allergies, asthma, and bronchitis; and can help people breathe easier.

I typically recommend combinations of both Cordyceps and reishi in capsule or liquid extract form—starting off with two capsules or one dropper full one to two times daily with the goal of getting at least 500 mg of each in a day.

Allergies to mushrooms are rare, but some people find them difficult to digest.

If you are passionate about mushrooms, you should discover the work of Paul Stamets, one of the leading mycologists in the world.[10] He is a great resource for learning more about the medicinal aspects of mushrooms and a personal friend of mine. Check him out.

Now that you are taking a good multivitamin, optimizing vitamin D and omega-3s—maybe using something for stress, energy, or a boost in immunity—you are well on your way! Only one step more: managing your physical body.

How we move determines how we live.

Studies abound showing that people who move their bodies on a daily basis live healthier, happier, more productive, and more vibrant lives. We want to figure out any way to do this that fits our lifestyle, resonates with our personality, and ultimately, is fun to do. Anything we enjoy becomes a *want to* not a *have to*.

MANAGING YOUR PHYSICAL BODY

WALK THE DOG

In order to walk the dog, you first have to get one. I understand that.

So what are you waiting for?

I like to walk my golden retriever, Cinnamon, every morning. Actually, she ends up walking me, but who's watching? There's something amazing about our morning ritual: first feeding Cinny and then watching her go directly from her dish to the front door, waiting for me with expectant eyes and wagging tail. On the off-hand chance that I don't get to walk her, the disappointment I witness is palpable.

I practice a form of walking meditation that I learned years ago and still use today (see "Go for a Breathwalk"). Accessing a state of focused relaxation in the midst of activity helps me to carry meditation into the real world. Sharing that experience with my doggie as the sun rises over the Catalina Mountains is something I eagerly look forward to and relish. Of course, she delights in it, too.

Walking the dog gets me moving every day and connects me with another living thing that is totally dependent on my care. My family and I enjoy her dependence on us to provide her with sustenance, comfort, and companionship (at least until we got the cat). Her unconditional love is felt powerfully. You've never lived until you've seen a dog smile. Do whatever it takes to make it happen.

Research shows that pets can instill a sense of fulfillment and well-being in people of all ages but especially the elderly.[1] Having a pet can lower blood pressure and feelings of depression.[2] It can speed recovery from a serious illness as well as raise levels of pet owners' self-esteem and security compared to those who don't have pets. Nursing homes have found their costs dropping when they've allowed pets to visit their patients. Stressed-out stockbrokers who have companion animals experience less anxiety. And the special bonus of having a dog to walk and play with is that it offers a continued excuse to keep moving.

If you do not have a dog, you can always become a volunteer walker at your local animal shelter. In addition to the animal-companionship benefits to your health, studies have found that burning just 500 extra calories per week can make a significant impact on all causes of mortality.[3] For an average person walking at 4 mph, approximately 100 calories are burned every 15 minutes. Walking your dog for just 15 minutes five days per week can decrease your risk of dying of anything, according to the Harvard Alumni Study.

Go walk a dog!

MOVE YOUR BODY EVERY DAY

Exercise is a key ingredient to achieving health. Not only does it help maintain normal weight by burning excess calories, but it can also modify the way your brain regulates hunger, in effect making you less susceptible to food cravings. Exercise prevents depression and boosts mood in healthy people. Like laughter, regular exercise can be a treatment for depression that is just as effective as medication, with less relapse. For all of those who know the secret of exercise, movement creates energy; it does not take it away. So exercise can also be quite effective for fatigue of any kind.

I am very interested in a form of activity called functional or integrative exercise. Integrative exercise concentrates on making movement fit into a routine by broadening the scope of activity to include the work of daily living, including things like gardening, household chores, grocery shopping, and yard work. Good data suggests that spending time doing more, preferably outside, can lead to just as many benefits as going to the gym.[1] When the healthiest old people are studied, most of them are not running marathons and attending aerobics classes; but almost everyone is continuing to do some kind of regular, functional activity to keep moving.

The biggest challenge I face as a clinician is that most individuals who do not exercise mistakenly think that they have to spend hours on end going to the gym to appreciate the benefits of extra activity. This is completely false.

Significant psychological and physiologic changes begin to occur in the body with as little as 75 to 90 minutes of walking per week (remember the Harvard Alumni Study). As a matter of fact, it is just as good, maybe even better, to break exercise apart in small chunks of time throughout the week as opposed to just one or two larger episodes.

So if you feel better gardening or mowing the lawn, walking your dog, landscaping your front yard, or having a major shop at Sam's Club, have at it.

It's good for you.

HIGH-INTENSITY INTERVAL TRAINING

When I do vigorous exercise, I like to do it in small bursts—one because I don't like to do it (being honest) and two, because as a busy physician and father of three, I don't have much time.

High-intensity interval training (HIIT) simply means doing a series of short bursts of intense exercise with short recovery breaks in between. I teach clients how to do this over a period of 20 to 30 minutes up to three times per week. I can't tell you how many times guests tell me they didn't get a chance to exercise because there wasn't an hour in their schedule to do it.

But they usually have 20 minutes sometime during the day.

Not only that, but HIIT keeps your focus by forcing you to change the intensity of the exercise intervals every minute. There is nothing worse than having to do exercise and being bored by it. Not so with HIIT.

It's not bad for efficiency either. A study of HIIT found that for every calorie expended during exercise, there was a nine-fold loss of subcutaneous body fat as compared to endurance trainers who road their bikes longer and even burned more calories.[1]

All I'm asking for is three times weekly for 20 minutes. If you want to do more or differently, go for it.

Obviously, there are some forms of exercise that work better than others. Finding a regimen that allows you to get it done while getting the best results is what I am looking to do and teach to my guests.

Give it a try.

You start by riding, walking, or using an elliptical machine at an intensity that you could do all day long. Make this really easy (don't worry, it'll change in a bit), and ride for two minutes at least. After the second minute, bump it up one level of intensity. I often describe this as the beginning of exercise, in that you've gone from something you could do forever to something that begins a sweat and makes you breathe a bit harder. Do this for one minute until you transition to the next level, which makes you breathe harder while still being able to carry on a conversation. The next minute and corresponding level, you're thinking about not talking, while the minute after that, your head is down and you're grinding it out. Do this for a minute and then go back to level two—the one right after "all day long"—and start over.

This comprises a set of four intervals of increasing intensity that you do three to five times during your workout. At the end, about the 18th or 23rd minute, you can really go for it by going from "head down, not talking" mode to what I call "give it all you've got" or "prayer mode," which is one additional level of intensity. When you finish with this minute, go back to "all day long" mode and pound your chest for a job well done. Do this as long as you like to cool down; you've earned it.

An important note: I don't recommend HIIT for people just recovering from an injury or beginning an exercise program for the first time. If you do begin this, start with moderate levels of intensity; you can always pick it up.

STRENGTH
TRAINING

I am a champion of a call to action known as Exercise Is Medicine, led by physicians and other practitioners in health care to emphasize physical activity as a prescription for the treatment of chronic disease. They have a website that offers great reference material to health practitioners who want to be more active in offering exercise counseling to their patients.

One of the core principles of integrative medicine is that all health practitioners (including doctors) should be models of health and healthy living. It does nothing but sabotage an individual's potential for success when his or her health-care provider is not modeling a healthy lifestyle.

It floored me when I heard news that 40 percent of primary care doctors and 36 percent of U.S. medical students do not meet the 2008 federal physical activity guidelines.[1] Consequently, it's not shocking that only 34 percent of American adults report having gotten any kind of exercise prescription during their last visit to a doctor.

That needs to change.

The federal guidelines speak about either exercising vigorously for a total of 150 minutes per week, doing 300 minutes of moderate-intensity aerobic activity, or an equivalent mix of each. You can refer to various websites to define these levels of intensity. Along with this, there is a recommendation to strengthen your muscles at least two days a week, doing exercises that work all the major muscle groups of your body (legs, hips, back, chest, abdomen, shoulders, and arms). This should be done using moderate to high intensity.

Working out with weights does so much more than making you look good and have tighter muscles. Strength training can stop, prevent, or even reverse both bone loss and muscle atrophy. Resistance training will also improve body mechanics and help with balance. It can boost mood by elevating endogenous opioids and other neurotransmitters that make us feel better. It can also stimulate metabolism by as high as 15 percent since more calories are required by the body to make and maintain muscle tissue as compared to fat. Strength training can benefit people of all ages and may be particularly important for those with chronic health conditions like arthritis, heart disease, or diabetes.

Remember, strength training does not have to be done solely with weights. You can use resistance bands; utilize your body weight as resistance by doing push-ups, leg lifts, sit-ups, and pull-ups; or do exercises like yoga and Pilates. You can also do functional exercises such as heavy gardening or landscaping that involves intense digging, shoveling, and lifting.

My preferred method of resistance training is weight lifting. Growing up as an athlete, I was introduced to weight training at an early age. At the time, it was a way to build muscle and stay strong. Now it has evolved to be so much more. Weight training has become a way for me to shut off my brain for a time and do nothing except be in my body. Silencing the chatter in my head is a beautiful thing. I don't socialize when I lift. It has become a wonderful meditation for me. If I work out with someone else, we usually have a singular focus. There's no messing around. But usually I do it alone.

I find that weight lifting allows me to adopt a certain physiology I call *victory mode*. I move my shoulders back with chest expanded and head and eyes forward, breathing fully and deeply. Moving my body this way gives me a feeling of invincibility—that I can do anything I set my mind to. It's nice to have that emotion coursing through me for 40 to 50 minutes a couple times a week. When I am done with a weight-training session, I always feel better than when I started. If I walk into the gym tired, angry, or feeling down, I usually leave with higher energy and in a good mood. Oftentimes, I thank myself and others for somehow finding a way to get me out of bed and to the gym.

Regarding where I work out, I find I like going somewhere else besides my home to do my weight training. I am less likely to be distracted at the gym. It is simply the pattern that has consistently worked the best for me.

The specifics of my workout follow the program Bill Phillips developed for his *Body for Life* book in the late 1990s.[2] At the time I read it, I was in medical school looking for a more efficient way to work out than the 8 to 10 hours weekly I was spending at the gym. My wife had just gotten pregnant, and I knew the windows of opportunity would significantly shrink in the near future, so I had to find a way to pack my exercise time into smaller increments. I have continued to do some form of the *Body for Life* exercise method for the past 13 years.

Why mess with a good thing?

Typically I will do two to three days of weight training weekly. In my 40s, I have found that I am not as intensely focused as before. My intention is to maintain what I have and not move backward as opposed to building lots of muscle.

I usually split up the major body parts, doing upper body and then skipping a day (when I will do a 20-minute HIIT session) and then doing lower body followed by another skipped day (HIIT), after which I will repeat the upper body session and then do my last HIIT of the week. I exercise six days a week and take one day off. The next week I will repeat the cycle except I will do two lower-body workouts with only one upper-body workout done mid-week.

My upper-body workout consists of two exercises each of biceps, triceps, chest, shoulders, and back. I will do six sets for each body part: five of one specific exercise followed by a different one for my burn-out session (as I describe in the next paragraph).

Sometimes I will use free weights, sometimes machines. My goal is to start out with very low intensity—just getting the motions down. I'll use a very light weight and get 12 repetitions done slowly and fluidly. I will wait a minute in between and then move up slightly in weight (usually by five- or ten-pound increments) and do the same exercise for ten repetitions. I will do the same thing for my third and fourth set, wait a minute in between, move up in weight, and then go for eight repetitions, followed by six. After another minute of waiting, I will then select the weight that I used to do eight repetitions and do my burnout sets by trying to get 12 reps with that weight. Immediately after the first set, I will then do what's called a super-set by moving to the next exercise without waiting, selecting a light weight, and then doing a different exercise than my first five for 12 repetitions. This is intense, and my muscles typically go to fatigue—hence the burnout.

The goal is to get to what Bill Phillips calls a "Level 10" experience, producing 100 percent focused intensity. Finishing this set should leave you with a fast heart rate, breathing deeply, and maybe even beginning to sweat. Working out this way makes your weight-training session aerobic in nature. It is definitely intense. After that body part is finished, I will then wait two minutes and move onto the next one. It usually takes me 50 minutes to finish an upper-body workout. Lower body takes less time since it only includes four exercises rather than five. I work on quadriceps, hamstrings, calves, and abdominals, following the same pattern I explained above.

The neat thing about working out this way is that you don't need a trainer or CDs to guide you through the process. You don't need all kinds of different exercise machines. I've seen people get amazing results with using a bench and a set of dumbbells.

I also love that it keeps my attention. My concentration tends to drift, and I can get easily distracted. Exercising this way is never boring. It is also the most intense workout I have ever tried for 40 to 50 minutes straight. There is no messing around.

You get in and get it done. That's the way I like it.

KNOW YOUR
TRIGGER POINTS

If you do any kind of strength training (which I recommend at least twice weekly), if you are under any kind of stress and have regular tension in your body, you have trigger points.

Trigger points are focal areas of tenderness, contraction, and irritability in muscles of the body that are injured or overworked. They often feel like lumps, knots, or ropes in the muscle. They were first identified decades ago by the research of two physicians, Doctors Janet Travell and David Simons. In their eyes, trigger points are the primary cause of pain in roughly 75 percent of situations and are at least part of the problem in most pain syndromes.[1]

I believe this to be true. I didn't know about trigger points until I went through my integrative medicine fellowship.

I know about them now.

Ten years ago during that same training program, I saw a woman with interstitial cystitis (IC). This is a difficult condition to treat, often called irritable bladder syndrome, that causes bladder pain and spasms, a feeling of urinary urgency along with the frequent need to urinate, pain and pressure in the lower abdomen, and difficult and uncomfortable sexual intercourse.

My patient had experienced these symptoms for three years and had been on several rounds of antibiotics (IC often gets confused with urinary infections) while enduring a battery of medical tests and procedures. Every conventional attempt was focused on trying to find the problem or treating it. Some of these tests were quite unpleasant, and several of them were expensive.

None of them worked until she came to the Arizona Center for Integrative Medicine and got trigger-point therapy from an old-time osteopathic physician named Dr. Harmon Myers.

Dr. Myers diagnosed her IC symptoms as directly caused by chronic trigger points in the floor of the pelvis and the inner aspect of her legs. Over a course of a few treatments involving gentle, mild stretches and holding her body in a particular position for no more than 90 seconds while the trigger points defused, he was able to completely take her symptoms away. Each treatment lasted about an hour.

This woman had not been pain free in several years. He cautioned her that the IC symptoms would return as these muscles tightened again, but simple stretches and self-massage could treat them effectively. She noticed the difference. As she developed discomfort, the stretches and massage therapy relieved it. So what did this doctor do that other doctors didn't or couldn't?

He treated her trigger points.

Even if these contribute to pain 25 percent of the time, we should know about them and learn how to how to treat them.

Sometimes you can do this yourself with massage, stretching, and passive positioning of your body. Any areas you have pain, look for trigger points by assessing with your fingers for areas of knotting or lumpiness. It typically feels like a rope in the muscle. If you have these and can get your hands on them, try applying sufficient pressure for about 60 seconds until the rope-like feeling softens. Using mentholated preparations (like Tiger Balm, Biofreeze, or Ben Gay) can also be helpful.

Good massage therapists, osteopaths, and chiropractors who effectively treat trigger points can be allies in your pursuit for health.

Seek them out.

MY TYPICAL DAY

My usual day starts somewhere between 4:30 and 6 A.M. Normally I don't need an alarm; the summer sun, my bladder, or an internal clock that is pretty reliable seems to wake me up.

I would like to think that I jump out of bed and start the day running, but at least half the time, I have an internal conversation with myself that goes something like this:

> *Okay, you're up. It's time to get up. You're not going to go back to sleep. What are you still doing in bed?!*
>
> *It's too damn early (especially at 4:30). Let me just lie here for the next 5 to 15 minutes and reevaluate the situation.*
>
> (Then, 5 to 15 minutes later . . .)
>
> *Okay, now it's <u>really</u> time to get up. You're wasting time. Get the #%&* up, Jim!*
>
> (This ultimately leads to . . .)

Lord, please help me get up. I don't think I can do this on my own. Please, God, help me get out of bed.

I can honestly say that I pray myself out of bed on a regular basis. The windows of opportunity for me to start the day the way I need to exist in the early morning, and yet, I have to say that it can still be a challenge getting started. I've found praying to be a pretty good formula; it rarely (if ever) has failed me. As a matter of fact, I don't think I can remember a time when it hasn't worked, which is why I do it so often.

Give it a try if you are so inclined.

Once I get out of bed, I will down the pint glass filled with water that is sitting on my nightstand and head to my closet to get dressed for the gym. I usually put on sweats or scrubs with a T-shirt and often a hoodie or light jacket (Arizona mornings are cool), a hat of some sort, and my hiking shoes. With my workout uniform donned, I say good-bye to the cat, who usually wants me to give her a morning scratch behind the ears, and then head to the gym.

Thankfully, the place where I work out is only five minutes away. I usually will grab a shot of espresso at home or on the way and take it with me; this ultimately becomes my water bottle. I have found that a small amount of espresso helps me wake up, gives me a better workout, and actually begins my thermogenesis without wiring me much.

When I get to the gym, I usually do a 20- to 30-minute aerobic session on the recumbent stationary bike or else I'll do a 50-minute strength-training workout, focusing on my upper body one day and my lower body two to three days later. I get at least two resistance-training workouts in most weeks (upper and lower body) and between three-to-four weekly aerobic sessions.

When I'm on the bike, I like to listen to music and read. Sometimes I'll watch ESPN on the TV, but usually it's reading time. The books I read range from biographies to nonfiction works on health or faith; but more often than not, I find myself escaping in books with a fantasy/adventure flavor.

Personally, the only window of opportunity for me to do formal exercise is in the early morning. My family is not yet awake. I'm a morning person, even with the occasional need for divine inspiration on the getting out of bed part, and the more I let the day progress without exercising, the more times I find myself letting it slip.

For me, doing hard things first starts with getting to the gym.

When I come home, my golden retriever, Cinnamon, is usually waiting for me to feed her with an excited tail wagging. While she is eating, I grab the leash. Once she's done inhaling her food, Cinny is primed and ready for a breathwalk. She will let me know if I'm stalling for whatever reason, pointing her way to the door and whining for me to get a move on.

We typically go for a 5- to 15-minute walk around our neighborhood, depending on how much time I have left before I need to get to work. I love walking in our community, saying hello to neighbors who have braved the morning, listening to birds, and watching wildlife skitter across the desert, waiting for the sun to peek out over the mountains.

Breathwalking starts my day off with mindfulness and an active meditation that I find hard to achieve sitting quietly. Besides, I have to walk the pooch.

Midway into my walk, I usually stop in the middle of a patch of communal desert just behind my house. I have fashioned a shrine there overlooking the Catalina Mountains. It's made of branches and saguaro spines on the ground in the shape of a heart, within which I've placed a circle of large stones and a bunch of smaller stones. I love to balance these smaller stones on top of each other to make a cairn sculpture. My kids have their own rock-balancing shrines around mine for when they come with me on my walks. They have put their names in rocks around my big circle within the branches, and they sometimes like to put their toys or action figures in the mix of stones.

Right now, there's a Boba Fett, a white tiger, a Dora, and a motorcyclist in the mix. It makes me smile.

In the stone and branch circle, I say a quick prayer, give the day to God, and ask for courage to make the day a masterpiece and serenity to accept what I can't control. Then, with a quick kiss to Cinny, who is waiting patiently for me to finish, I find my way back home. During this short walk, I launch into a quick gratitude practice, saying thank you for all the things I am grateful for right now, as well as anything I can think of that has happened over the past couple of days. I also think about things I want to manifest in my future, visualizing them occuring and giving thanks that they've taken place, expecting that they have already done so. I call this practice the *gratitude spiral*.

Taken together, this is what I call the Big Three:

1.   Get to the gym.

2.   Go for a breathwalk.

3.   Get grateful and give the day to God.

I do these most days.

When I get home, it's usually hop in the shower, do my daily hygiene, get dressed for work, make breakfast, and help my wife, Sara, get the kids ready for the day. Most of the time, I help see them on their school bus. Sometimes I take Kyle early, where he can run laps around the school track in a club called Milers. He earns a medal for every five miles he runs. I encourage him to do this. Summertime is a bit more lax. Usually the kids sleep in except for my youngest, who is a morning person like me. Ava always gets a hug and a kiss before work.

Miraval is about 15 minutes away. I start my drive with breathing exercises, listen to instrumental music (usually soundtracks to movies), and maybe try to touch base with friends or relatives via the phone.

The Integrative Wellness Center is five minutes away from the parking lot. I breathwalk my way there, the Catalina mountains serving as my morning backdrop. It's a great way to get to work and commit my day to serving God and the guests I see.

My office is a neat space. When I get in, I put on soothing music via my iPod. I've been using an album called *The Drone* as background music for when I see guests and do other work in the office. It is a recording of C and G notes played simultaneously. This tone is described musically as the interval of the perfect fifth. The sound it offers provides a gentle, harmonic background to my day, whatever it may look like. It keeps me calm.

Usually my work day involves some form of teaching, either in a classroom setting or small seminar format. I see guests for one-on-one consultations, do a fair amount of writing, and answer e-mails and phone calls from past guests wanting to stay in touch. I also reply to a number of media requests regarding health-related material, especially from an integrative medicine perspective.

Being the medical director of the Integrative Wellness Program also provides me with opportunities to meet with the various practitioners Miraval has to offer. This is the *interactive* part of the program. As Dr. Weil has said, "A good integrative physician learns how to create therapeutic marriages between patients and practitioners." Understanding an individual's needs allows me to refer guests to the various experts, specialists, and practitioners on the Miraval campus. Whether that might include dietary intervention, exercise prescriptions, acupuncture, massage, shamanic healing, meditation, or other mind-body therapies, by developing relationships with these experts, I can help guide guests to a set of experiences that may offer them the best chance to find healing.

A nice perk is being on the other side of the healing encounter. I get to experience everything Miraval has to offer: from yoga and the outdoor adventure challenge courses to the various spa services available. Having a hands-on feel for therapies and the specific practitioners that offer them allows me to make that marriage of services work best to suit an individual's needs.

I haven't gotten to everything offered here at Miraval, but I'm working on it.

I also meet with Dr. Weil on a weekly basis to go over guests I have seen, potentially asking him for advice about recommendations for them or how he might address a certain situation. He has a world of knowledge and experience that I want to have access to, and I appreciate this kind of forum. We talk about upcoming projects and what might be going on in the integrative medicine world. We also chat about food, books, and movies and have the occasional political conversation. He continues to serve as a mentor, advising me on the work I do as a physician and healer, while also trying to keep me in line.

He tries.

He is my very good friend.

I usually get home in the early evening. If the kids are going somewhere—baseball practice, swimming, gymnastics, or dance—we typically make a quick dinner and get where we need to be. Sometimes Sara and I split up and chauffeur the kids to different places. We try to stay together as much as possible.

At least three of the seven days, we make a concerted effort to eat at the dinner table. I love to cook and find that it's a great way to unwind from a busy day at work. Chopping vegetables, making salad dressings and sauces, stir-frying, or grilling all can be remarkably relaxing and creative at the same time. There is nothing better than to sit down together as a family and have a great meal. We like to play games during dinner like "Roses and Thorns" (got that one from President Obama and the First Lady) or the ABC game, where we go around creating words with one, two, or three letters from the alphabet—*amazing, aerobic acrobats* or *belligerent, brown basilisks*—and the like (the kids always say I'm a geek for the words I use). Fun stuff.

Homework and baths come after and then maybe some movie time if there are any hours left in the day. Sometimes the kids and I might play on the Wii. I love bowling and tennis; they love "Mario Kart." We can get into some serious competitions, my kids and me. Sara is the referee.

Bedtime happens at 8:30 for my daughter, where she usually ends up falling asleep on the couch and I have to take her to her room upstairs. The boys will get to bed around 9 or 9:15. Knowing that I will be getting up at the crack of dawn, I'm often right behind them. I turn in no later than 10, maybe even 9:30 after doing my evening hygiene.

I'm pretty good with seven hours of sleep. I can get by with six but not too frequently. Sleeping longer than eight hours often gives me a backache and leaves me sluggish. I haven't slept in for quite some time. I typically end the day with a good book (if I can), which helps me drift right to sleep.

The pint glass of water is waiting on the nightstand for my morning chug, and this begins the process for tomorrow's rituals of the day.

Having found ways to move and doing it regularly, being in touch with your trigger points, and understanding how to recognize when your body is working for you and when it is out of balance . . . we find ourselves at the end of our journey.

That is exactly what I picture the concept of wellness to be: where health is the *destination* and wellness is the *journey.* Health is ultimately the place you are trying to get to, and once you arrive, you want to stay there. Unfortunately, health is shifty—it's like the island in the TV series *Lost,* constantly moving, changing, and knocking you off balance.

If wellness is the journey, think of it as everything we use to get us to our destination: it's the vehicle and the fuel; the map and the GPS; the spare tire and the jack. But the journey also includes the people we meet, the conversations we have, the music we listen to, and the food and drink we share. The journey is filled with memories and experiences gathered as we go.

And what we discover is that the journey is where we find all the joy. It is not necessarily the achievement of the goal that counts as opposed to what we've discovered along the way. It is the learning, the doing, the practicing, the uncertainty, the struggle, falling down and getting up, and the process of living throughout that makes our voyage so rewarding. Think of these wellness strategies as pieces along your journey. Experiment with them. Find ones that work; discard ones that don't. And through it all, remember to appreciate the process and be present wherever you are along the way. Here's to the journey!

AFTERWORD

Hopefully you've found this book to be a quick and easy read. That was my goal. Now it's time to put it all together.

As you go through these ideas and approaches to health, take a look at which ones speak to your heart and your gut, just as much as your head. If you have found two or three health tips that resonate with you and that you are willing to try, I suggest that you work hard practicing them for the next three months.

Most of us can get our heads around a time period of 12 weeks. It's not so long that we get too distracted, lose track, or forget, but it is a long enough time to notice a difference once we're finished.

During this three-month period, come up for air every two weeks and evaluate how things are going. You might notice subtle changes between two and four weeks; certainly, you should detect something at eight weeks. (Dr. Weil wrote about these changes in his book, *8 Weeks to Optimum Health.*[1]) I want you to keep an intense focus over another four weeks for a total span of three months. Remember, I like threes.

After this time, if you have noticed an improvement in your health—more energy, less pain, a better body, less depression, more confidence, and a sense of fulfillment—then you deserve big congratulations. You've just become extraordinary. Keep it up!

Add to your wellness strategies as you see fit. Check off your goals and accomplishments from your journal and vision board. When you're done, give yourself a smile of satisfaction, do a happy dance, reward yourself with something nice, and then start over with a new dream.

Health is like a garden. If we don't tend it, weeds grow and strangle our roses. Our garden should be lush and beautiful. Complacency makes weeds.

We should remember the wisdom of a classic fairy tale and film, *The Princess Bride,* when the six-fingered man utters these famous words to Prince Humperdinck on the eve of his wedding: "If you don't have your health, you don't have anything!"[2]

May you be on your way to better health and wellness.

By the way, if you would like to share a certain health rule or strategy that I have not included, especially ones that you have found particularly useful, please e-mail me at the following website: **www .drjimnicolai.com**.

Thanks for the tip.

— **Dr. Jim Nicolai**
Miraval Resort and Spa, Tucson

APPENDIXES

THE ANTI-INFLAMMATORY DIET

This is a summary of the specifics of a diet intended to prevent inappropriate inflammation. It is reprinted with permission by **www .drweil.com**. The Anti-Inflammatory Diet is not a diet in the popular sense; it is not intended as a weight-loss program (although people can and do lose weight on it), and neither is it an eating plan to stay on for a limited period of time. Rather, it is way of selecting and preparing foods based on scientific knowledge of how they can help your body maintain optimum health. Along with influencing inflammation, this diet will provide steady energy and ample vitamins, minerals, essential fatty acids, dietary fiber, and protective phytonutrients. You can also adapt your existing recipes according to these anti-inflammatory diet principles:

General Diet Tips

- Aim for variety.
- Include as much fresh food as possible.
- Minimize your consumption of processed foods and fast food.
- Eat an abundance of fruits and vegetables.

Caloric Intake

- Most adults need to consume between 2,000 and 3,000 calories a day.
- Women and smaller, less active people need fewer calories.
- Men and bigger, more active people need more calories.
- If you are eating the appropriate number of calories for your level of activity, your weight should not fluctuate greatly.
- The distribution of calories you take in should be as follows: 40 to 50 percent from carbohydrates, 30 percent from fat, and 20 to 30 percent from protein.
- Try to include carbohydrates, fat, and protein at each meal.

Carbohydrates

- On a 2,000-calorie-a-day diet, adult women should consume between 160 to 200 grams of carbohydrates a day.

- Adult men should consume between 240 to 300 grams of carbohydrates a day.

- The majority of this should be in the form of less-refined, less-processed foods with a low glycemic load.

- Reduce your consumption of foods made with wheat flour and sugar, especially bread and most packaged snack foods (including chips and pretzels).

- Eat more whole grains such as brown rice and bulgur wheat, in which the grain is intact or in a few large pieces. These are preferable to whole wheat flour products, which have roughly the same glycemic index as white-flour products.

- Eat more beans, winter squashes, and sweet potatoes.

- Cook pasta al dente, and eat it in moderation.

- Avoid products made with high-fructose corn syrup.

Fat

- On a 2,000-calorie-a-day diet, 600 calories can come from fat—that is, about 67 grams. This should be in a ratio of 1:2:1 of saturated to monounsaturated to polyunsaturated fat.

- Reduce your intake of saturated fat by eating less butter, cream, high-fat cheese, chicken with skin and fatty meats, and products made with palm kernel oil.

- Use extra-virgin olive oil as your main cooking oil. If you want a neutral-tasting oil, use expeller-pressed, organic canola oil. Organic, high-oleic, expeller-pressed versions of sunflower and safflower oil are also acceptable.

- Avoid regular safflower and sunflower oils, corn oil, cottonseed oil, and mixed vegetable oils.

- Strictly avoid margarine and vegetable shortening and all products listing them as ingredients. Strictly avoid all products made with partially hydrogenated oils of any kind. Include in your diet avocados and nuts, especially walnuts, cashews, almonds, and nut butters made from these nuts.

- For omega-3 fatty acids, eat salmon (preferably fresh or frozen wild or canned sockeye), sardines packed in water or olive oil, herring, and black cod (sablefish, butterfish); omega-3 fortified eggs; hemp seeds and flaxseeds (preferably freshly ground); or take a fish oil supplement (look for products that provide both EPA and DHA in a convenient daily dosage of two to three grams).

Protein

- On a 2,000-calorie-a-day diet, your daily intake of protein should be between 80 and 120 grams. Eat less protein if you have liver or kidney problems, allergies, or autoimmune disease.

- Decrease your consumption of animal protein except for fish and high-quality natural cheese and yogurt.

- Eat more vegetable protein, especially from beans in general and soybeans in particular. Become familiar with the range of whole-soy foods available, and find ones you like.

Fiber

- Try to eat 40 grams of fiber a day. You can achieve this by increasing your consumption of fruit, especially berries, vegetables (especially beans), and whole grains.

- Ready-made cereals can be good fiber sources, but read labels to make sure they give you at least four and preferably five grams of bran per one-ounce serving.

Phytonutrients

- To get maximum natural protection against age-related diseases (including cardiovascular disease, cancer, and neurodegenerative disease) as well as against environmental toxicity, eat a variety of fruits, vegetables, and mushrooms.

- Choose fruits and vegetables from all parts of the color spectrum, especially berries, tomatoes, orange and yellow fruits, and dark, leafy greens.

- Choose organic produce whenever possible. Learn which conventionally grown crops are most likely to carry pesticide residues and avoid them.

- Eat cruciferous (cabbage-family) vegetables regularly.

- Include soy foods in your diet.

- Drink tea instead of coffee, especially good-quality white, green, or oolong tea.

- If you drink alcohol, use red wine preferentially.

- Enjoy plain dark chocolate in moderation (with a minimum cocoa content of 70 percent).

Vitamins and Minerals

- The best way to obtain all of your daily vitamins, minerals, and micronutrients is by eating a diet high in fresh foods, with an abundance of fruits and vegetables. In addition, supplement your diet with the following antioxidant cocktail:

- Vitamin C, 200 milligrams a day.

- Vitamin E, 400 IU of natural mixed tocopherols (d-alpha-tocopherol with other tocopherols, or better, a minimum of 80 milligrams of natural mixed tocopherols and tocotrienols).

- Selenium, 200 micrograms of an organic (yeast-bound) form.

- Mixed carotenoids, 10,000 to 15,000 IU daily.

- The antioxidants can be most conveniently taken as part of a daily multivitamin/multimineral supplement that also provides at least 400 micrograms of folic acid and 2,000 IU of vitamin D. It should contain no iron (unless you are a female and having regular menstrual periods) and no preformed vitamin A (retinol). Take these supplements with your largest meal.

- Women should take supplemental calcium, preferably as calcium citrate, 500 to 700 milligrams a day, depending on their dietary intake of this mineral. Men should avoid supplemental calcium.

Other Dietary Supplements

- If you are not eating oily fish at least twice a week, take supplemental fish oil in capsule or liquid form (two to three grams a day of a product containing both EPA and

DHA). Look for molecularly distilled products certified to be free of heavy metals and other contaminants.

- Talk to your doctor about going on low-dose aspirin therapy, one or two baby aspirins a day (81 or 162 milligrams).

- If you are not regularly eating ginger and turmeric, consider taking these in supplemental form.

- Add coQ10 to your daily regimen: 60 to 100 milligrams of a soft-gel form taken with your largest meal.

- If you are prone to metabolic syndrome, take alpha-lipoic acid, 100 to 400 milligrams a day.

Water

- Drink pure water, or drinks that are mostly water (tea, very-diluted fruit juice, sparkling water with lemon) throughout the day.

- Use bottled water or get a home water purifier if your tap water tastes of chlorine or other contaminants or if you live in an area where the water is known or suspected to be contaminated.

DIETARY SUPPLEMENTS

I recommend and personally use Weil Lifestyle brand vitamins. They are based on scientifically validated formulas and are continuously overseen by Dr. Weil and his team of experts, in part due to his dissatisfaction with what has been previously available in the marketplace. These vitamins are available at Miraval Resorts Arizona as well as on Dr. Weil's website. Go to **www.drweil.com** and click on "Weil Nutritional Supplements." Below are general guidelines for choosing from the wide array of multivitamin, multi-mineral products available now on the market. There are many reasonable combinations of ingredients but just as many carelessly formulated that may not offer sound nutrition or complete safety. Also below is Dr. Weil's complete daily antioxidant and multivitamin/mineral formula, which I consider to be the basic requirement as insurance against gaps in the diet.

Please note that all of Dr. Weil's after-tax profits from royalties from sales of Weil Lifestyle, LLC, retail products go directly to the Weil Foundation. The Weil Foundation is an independent 501(c)(3) organization dedicated to supporting integrative medicine through training, education, and research. This is one of the many reasons why I recommend and use these products, because I am a passionate supporter of the work Dr. Weil is doing in promoting the advancement of integrative medicine.

I recommend taking a daily multivitamin, multi-mineral product that meets the following recommendations:

- Does not contain any preformed vitamin A (retinol/retinol palmitate).

- Includes a mixture of carotenoids, not just beta carotene. This should include lutein and lycopene, as well as other members of this family of antioxidant pigments like astaxanthin and zeaxanthin.

- It should provide vitamin E as mixed, natural tocopherols, not just d-alpha-tocopherol or worse, synthetic dl-alpha-tocopherol. Better-quality products will also provide mixed tocotrienols, the other components of the natural vitamin E complex.

- 50 milligrams each of most B vitamins, except for folic acid (at least 400 micrograms) and vitamin B12 (at least 50 micrograms).

- It need not contain much more than 200 to 250 milligrams of vitamin C, which research suggests is all the human body can use in a day.

- Provides at least 1,000 IU of vitamin D. Note: You will need to take additional vitamin D to get the recommended daily intake of 2,000 IU.

- Does not contain iron, unless you are a menstruating woman, are pregnant, or have documented iron-deficiency anemia.

- Includes no more than 200 micrograms of selenium, a key-antioxidant mineral, preferably in its yeast-bound form.

- It should provide some calcium as calcium citrate, though it is not recommended that men supplement with any calcium. (Several studies suggest increased calcium intake may be a risk factor for prostate cancer in men.) Women should probably get no more than 500 to 700 mg daily from supplements and men no more than 500 mg from all sources.

A product that meets all of the above recommendations will probably require taking more than one pill or capsule. I usually recommend taking water-soluble vitamins separate from fat-soluble ones. You can take your multivitamins any time of day, but always do so with a full stomach to avoid indigestion. Fat-soluble vitamins like vitamin E and the carotenoids need fat to be absorbed optimally.

Any product is most efficient and easily taken once daily.

Formula for Dr. Weil Daily Antioxidant, Multivitamin-multi-mineral (2 vegetarian tablets, 1 vegetarian capsule)

d-alpha tocopherol: 67 mg (~ 100 IU)
d-beta tocopherol: 2.25 mg
d-gammatocopherol: 80 mg
d- delta tocopherol: 18 mg
d-alpha tocopherol: 5 mg
d-beta tocotrienols: 0.6 mg
d-gamma tocotrienols: 9 mg
d-delta tocotrienols: 2.4 mg
selenium (yeast bound): 200 mcg
coenzyme Q-10: 30 mg
alpha carotene: 1 mg
astaxanthin: 750 mcg
vitamin A (as beta carotene): 15,000 IU
gamma carotene: 132 mcg
lutein: 5 mg
zeaxanthin: 300 mcg
lycopene: 10 mg
phytoene: 800 mcg

phytofluene: 800 mcg
vitamin D (as cholecalciferol): 1–2,000 IU
vitamin C: 250 mg
thiamine: 50 mg
riboflavin: 50 mg
niacin (as niacinamide, B3): 50 mg
vitamin B6 (pyridoxine HCl): 50 mg
vitamin B12: 50 mcg
folate (as folic acid): 400 mcg
biotin (as d-biotin): 100 mcg
pantothenic acid (as d-calcium pantothenate): 50 mg
calcium (as calcium citrate): 60 mg
iodine (source: kelp): 150 mcg
magnesium (as magnesium citrate): 30 mg
zinc15: mg
copper: 1.5 mg
manganese: 1 mg
chromium: 200 mcg
molybdenum: 75 mcg
potassium: 1 mg
choline: 50 mg
citrus bioflavonoids (as a complex): 40 mg
inositol: 50 mg
PABA: 50 mg
rutin: 40 mg
silicon (as silicon dioxide): 2 mg
sulphur (as MSM): 5 mg
vanadium: 10 mcg

A NOTE ON INTEGRATIVE MEDICINE

Integrative medicine is healing-oriented medicine that takes account of the whole person (body, mind, and spirit), including all aspects of lifestyle. It emphasizes the practitioner-patient relationship and makes use of all appropriate therapies, both conventional and alternative.

Dr. Weil founded and continues to direct the University of Arizona's Program in Integrative Medicine, which was recently designated as a Center of Excellence and is now known as the Arizona Center for Integrative Medicine, to lead a transformation in health care by educating and supporting a community of professionals who are expert in the principles and practice of this new system.

Since its inception, the Arizona Center for Integrative Medicine (AzCIM) has focused its efforts on three domains: education, clinical care, and research—with the primary emphasis on education.

1. *Education.* The center offers a broad range of educational opportunities for health-care professionals with an interest in learning and practicing the principles of integrative medicine. The majority of the center's educational offerings are online, including the flagship program: The Fellowship in Integrative Medicine.

2. *Clinical Care.* The Arizona Center for Integrative Medicine has two clinical locations at the University of Arizona, specializing in creating integrative treatment plans for patients with medical conditions ranging from cancer to chronic conditions, such as diabetes and heart disease, as well as offering preventative care.

3. *Research.* The center's goal is to contribute rigorous scientific research on the integration of complementary and alternative therapies with conventional methods. They focus on three areas: educational research, corporate health research, and methods to study clinical outcomes in integrative medicine.

The Arizona Center for Integrative Medicine has been the leading provider of integrative medical education worldwide. They have developed the first and most comprehensive academic curriculum, in addition to creating the first family medicine-integrative medicine combined residency program in the United States. AzCIM has trained over 500 fellows, many of whom are now leaders in integrative medicine across the country and the world. Alumni include medical practitioners from 45 states, as well as Canada, Japan, Korea, Israel, United Arab Emirates, the U.S. Virgin Islands, and Puerto Rico. Faculty and graduates have contributed to the field by writing leading textbooks on integrative medicine, as well as numerous textbook chapters and articles. AzCIM has also been the co-founder of the Consortium of Academic Health Centers for Integrative Medicine—currently an association of 50 academic centers with their deans from leading medical programs like Duke, Harvard, Georgetown, University of California–San Francisco, and other highly esteemed medical centers and their affiliate institutions.

For more information about AZCIM, visit **www.integrative medicine.arizona.edu**.

SUGGESTED READING, RESOURCES, AND PRODUCTS

Books

Bell, Rob. *Velvet Elvis: Repainting the Christian Faith* (Grand Rapids, MI: Zondervan, 2005).

———. *Sex God: Exploring the Endless Connections between Sexuality and Spirituality* (Grand Rapids, MI: Zondervan, 2008).

———. *Love Wins: A Book about Heaven, Hell, and the Fate of Every Person Who Ever Lived* (New York: HarperOne, 2011).

Campbell, Joseph. *The Hero with a Thousand Faces,* New World Library, third edition (New York: Pantheon Books, 2008).

Childre, Doc, and Howard Martin, with Donna Beech. *The HeartMath Solution: The Institute of HeartMath's Revolutionary Program for Engaging the Power of Heart intelligence* (San Francisco, CA: HarperCollins, 2000).

Childre, Doc, and Deborah Rozman. *Transforming Stress: The HeartMath Solution for Relieving Worry, Fatigue, and Tension* (Oakland, CA: New Harbinger Publications, 2005).

Goleman, Daniel. *Emotional Intelligence: Why It Can Matter More than IQ* (New York: Bantam, 1995).

Gonzalez-Wippler, Migene. *Keys to the Kingdom: Jesus and the Mystic Kabbalah* (St. Paul, MN: Llewellyn Publications, 2004).

Gurgevich, Steven. *Hypnosis House Call: A Complete Course in Mind-Body Healing* (New York, Sterling Publishing, 2010).

Heber, David. *What Color Is Your Diet?* (New York: HarperCollins, 2001).

Holick, Michael. *The Vitamin D Solution: A 3-Step Strategy to Cure Our Most Common Health Problem* (New York: Hudson Street Press, 2010).

Holtz, Lou. *Winning Every Day: The Game Plan for Success* (New York: Harper Collins, 1998).

Miraval. *Mindful Eating* (Carlsbad, CA: Hay House, 2012).

Phillips, Bill, and Mike D'Orso. *Body for Life* (New York: Harper Collins, 1999).

Phillips, Bill. *Transformation: The Mindset You Need. The Body You Want. The Life You Deserve.* (Los Angeles, CA: T-Media, 2011).

Pollan, Michael. *Food Rules: An Eater's Manual* (New York: Penguin, 2009).

Pressfield, Steven. *The War of Art: Break Through the Blocks and Win Your Inner Creative Battles* (New York: Grand Central Publishing, 2003).

———. *Do the Work! Overcome Resistance and Get Out of Your Own Way* (The Domino Project, 2011)

———. *The Warrior Ethos* (New York: Black Irish Entertainment, 2011).

Robbins, Anthony. *Unlimited Power: The New Science of Personal Achievement* (New York, Free Press, 1986).

———. *Awaken the Giant Within: How to Take Immediate Control of Your Mental, Emotional, Physical and Financial Destiny* (New York: Free Press, 1992).

Singh Khalsa, Gurucharan, and Yogi Bhajan. *Breathwalk: Breathing Your Way to a Revitalized Body, Mind and Spirit* (New York: Broadway Books, 2000).

Sylvia, Claire, with William Novak. *A Change of Heart: A Memoir* (New York: Little, Brown and Company, 1997).

Weil, Andrew. *Spontaneous Happiness* (New York: Little, Brown and Company, 2011).

———. *Natural Health, Natural Medicine: The Complete Guide to Wellness and Self-Care for Optimum Health,* rev. ed. (Boston, MA: Houghton Mifflin, 2004)

———. *8 weeks to Optimum Health: A Proven Program for Taking Full Advantage of Your Body's Natural Healing Power,* rev. ed. (New York: Ballantine, 2006)

———. *Healthy Aging: A Lifelong Guide to Your Physical and Spiritual Well-Being* (New York: Knopf, 2005).

———. *Spontaneous Healing: How to Discover and Enhance Your Body's Natural Ability to Maintain and Heal Itself* (New York: Ballantine Books, 2000).

———. *Eating for Optimum Health: The Essential Guide to Bringing Health and Pleasure Back to Eating* (New York: HarperCollins, 2001).

Wilcox, Bradley, D. Craig Wilcox, and Makota Suzuki, *The Okinawa Program: How the World's Longest-Lived People Achieve Everlasting Health—and How You Can Too* (New York: Three Rivers Press, 2002).

Websites

Academy for Guided Imagery: **www.acadgi.com**

American Music Therapy Association: **www.musictherapy.org**

Anthony Robbins: **www.tonyrobbins.com**

The Arizona Center for Integrative Medicine: **www.AzCIM.org**

Bill Phillips : **www.transformation.com**

Body-*for*-Life: **www.Bodyforlife.com**

Dr. Andrew Weil: **www.drweil.com**

Exercise Is Medicine: **www.exerciseismedicine.org**

Federal Exercise Guidelines: **www.cdc.gov/physicalactivity/everyone/guidelines/index.html**

Laughter Clubs: **www.laughteryoga.org**

Molly Stranahan: **www.mollystranahan.com**

Nooma videos: **www.nooma.com**

Rob Bell: **www.robbell.com**

Steve Gurgevich: **www.tranceformation.com**

Steven Pressfield: **www.stevenpressfield.com**

Tucson Symphony Orchestra: **www.tucsonsymphony.org**

Audio Programs

Harold Moses, "The Drone," Crucible Sound, Inc., 2000.

Tony Robbins, "Personal Power II: The Driving Force." Robbins Research International, Inc. (1996)

————. "Power Talk! Strategies for Lifelong Success. N.A.P.I. Publishing; Unabridged edition (2002).

————. "Get the Edge: A 7-Day Program To Transform Your Life." Guthy-Renker, 2000.

Andrew Weil, "Breathing: The Master Key to Self-Healing," Sounds True audio edition, 1999.

————. "Sound Body, Sound Mind." Rhino, 2005.

Andrew Weil and Joshua Leeds, "Relax and De-Stress." Sounds True, 2009.

————. "Deep Calm." Sounds True, 2009.

Andrew Weil and Kemba Arem. "Vibrational Sound Healing." Sounds True, 2010.

Video Programs

Rob Bell, "Nooma—Breathe," Flannel, 2006.

Andrew Weil, "Dr. Andrew Weil's Health Aging: A Guide to Achieving Lifelong Health and Happiness From America's Most Trusted Physician." Acacia, 2006.

————. "Dr. Andrew Weil's Guide to Eating Well." Acacia, 2007.

Products

As stated previously, I recommend and use Weil Lifestyle brand vitamins from DrWeil.com. Other dietary supplements, products, and services that align with my recommendations in this book include the following.

Medicinal Mushroom Products

This company makes extracts of Cordyceps and reishi, called CordyChi that I recommend, along with immune system–boosting extracts called Host Defense.

Fungi Perfecti
P.O. Box 7634
Olympia, Washington 98507
800-780-9126
www.fungi.com

I periodically take medicinal mushroom extracts of Cordyceps and reishi called LifeShield Breathe and LifeShield Immunity available from:

New Chapter Company
22 High Street
Brattleboro, Vermont 05301
800-543-7279
www.newchapter.com

Fish Oil Supplements

Nordic Naturals
94 Hanger Way
Watsonville, California 96076
800-662-2544
www.nordicnaturals.com

Herbs with Anti-inflammatory Properties

For supercritical extracts of ginger and turmeric, plant-based extracts of holy basil, and the combination herbal anti-inflammatory product Zyflamend:

New Chapter Company
22 High Street
Brattleboro, Vermont 05301
800-543-7279
www.newchapter.com

Matcha and Other Fine Teas

Matcha and More
4901 W. Warick
Chicago, Illinois 60641
877-534-0505
www.matchaandmore.com

In Pursuit of Tea
1435 Fourth Street
Berkely, California 94710
866-878-3832 x 5
www.inpursuitoftea.com

Seafood and Omega-3 Fatty Acid–Rich Fish

Vital Choice Wild Seafood & Organics
2460 Salashan Loop Road
Ferndale, Washington 98248
800-608-4825
www.vitalchoice.com

Water Purifiers

Kinetico Home Water Systems
10845 Kinsman Road
Newbury, Ohio 44065
800-944-9283
www.kinetico.com

ENDNOTES

Preface

1. For anyone who is a raving *Star Wars* fan like me, you can read more about carbon freezing (yes, this is fantasy) from Wookiepedia—the Star Wars Wiki website: **www.starwars.wikia.com/wiki/Carbon_freezing**.

Introduction

1. Most of my statistical information came from Coach Wooden's official website: **www.coachwooden.com**. He shares his seven-point credo in a video on this website; however, I first heard about the story from an interview John Wooden did with Tony Robbins in 1992, recorded from one of his Power Talk! sessions.

Dream Big

1. Steven Pressfield, *Gates of Fire.* Random House Digital, Inc., September 27, 2005.

2. Steven Pressfield, *Do the Work!* The Domino Project, 2011.

Set Health Goals

1. Paul J. Meyer describes the characteristics of SMART goals in his book, *Attitude Is Everything: If You Want to Succeed Above and Beyond,* from the Leading Edge Publishing Company (2006).

2. I first read about the concept of transformational vocabulary in Tony Robbins' book *Awaken the Giant Within.* He has talked about this in subsequent audio recordings and in his seminars.

Keep a Journal

1. This is another quote from Tony Robbins (**www.tonyrobbins.com**).

The Map and the Mind-Set

1. I heard that this saying comes from Thomas Edison and validated it through several websites. There are great quotes from his official website: **www.thomasedison.com**.

2. For more information on this idea, visit Tony Robbins's website: **www.tonyrobbins.com**.

Role Models and Archetypes

1. This was first depicted by Joseph Campbell in his 1949 classic, *The Hero with a Thousand Faces* (New World Library, third edition, 2008). You can get more information about Joseph Campbell's work on his official website: **www.jcf.org**.

Take a Day Off

1. This is specifically described in *Body for Life* by Bill Phillips, pages 91–93.

Follow Your Heart

1. To learn more about the research and scientifically validated work done at the Institute of HeartMath, visit the following website: **www.heartmath.org**. To access further information about using HeartMath products to improve health and performance, visit their website at **www.heartmath.com**.

2. This is documented in a memoir called *A Change of Heart* by Claire Sylvia (Boston, MA: Little, Brown and Company, 1998).

Listen to the Whisper

1. This appears in the Bible—1 Kings 19:11–13 according to the New International Version (NIV) as follows:

   The LORD said, "Go out and stand on the mountain in the presence of the LORD, for the LORD is about to pass by."
   Then a great and powerful wind tore the mountains apart and shattered the rocks before the LORD, but the LORD was not in the wind. After the wind there was an earthquake, but the LORD was not in the earthquake. After the earthquake came a fire, but the LORD was not in the fire. And after the fire came a gentle whisper. When Elijah heard it, he pulled his cloak over his face and went out and stood at the mouth of the cave.
   Then a voice said to him, "What are you doing here, Elijah?"

Believe in Magic

1. This appears in *Spontaneous Healing* by Andrew Weil (New York: Ballantine, 2000).

Give the Day to God

1. The version of the Lord's Prayer that I use comes from a book by Migene Gonzalez-Wippler called *Keys to the Kingdom: Jesus and the Mystic Kabbalah.*

2. Rob Bell describes his interpretation of the ancient Hebrew word for God in a video called *Breathe* (Nooma, 2006).

Get into Nature

1. I found this quote within my reading of a piece from Neil Peart's website—**www.neilpeart.net**—recommending one of Aldous Huxley's treasured books: *After Many Summers Dies the Swan.*

2.   For further information on the work of Nancy Etcoff, Ph.D., and the Home Ecology of Flowers study see the following press release: **http://community.passiongrowers.com/wp-content/uploads/2010/08/flowersinthehome1017061.pdf**.

Give to Live

1.   This interesting information came from, of all places, Wikipedia, which helped with the biblical references. See **http://en.wikipedia.org/wiki/Tithe**. I also referenced First Fruits using the website: **http://en.wikipedia.org/wiki/First_fruits**.

2.   Grateful acknowledgment to Molly L. Stranahan, Psy.D., for permission to reprint her Strategy of Generosity excerpt. You can learn more about Molly Stranahan and the work she does on her website at: **www.mollystranahan.com**.

Go for a Breathwalk

1.   Written about by Yogi Bhajan, Ph.D., and Guruchan Singh Khalsa, Ph.D., in their book *Breathwalk* (New York: Broadway Books, 2000). There is also a companion cassette tape set entitled *Breathwalks* made by the same authors. It is difficult to obtain due to being out of circulation, but it has specific audio recordings along with a 32-page guidebook to take you through particular breathwalking patterns. For more information, you can also visit the Kundalini Research Institute at: **www.kundaliniresearchinstitute.org/breathwalk/welcome.html**.

Swing and a Prayer

1.   I found much of the information about Gayle King's experience from Oprah Winfrey's website: **www.oprah.com/oprahshow/Letters-to-Oprah**.

2.   Grateful acknowledgment to Kim Granderson for permission to reprint her Swing and a Prayer experience.

Laugh Often

1.   Much of the amazing work that Dr. Kataria and his wife continue to do with laughter is available on their website: **www.laughteryoga.org**.

Find a Friend in a Pet

1. One particular study comes from the University of Cambridge by J. Serpell, entitled "Beneficial effects of pet ownership on some aspects of human health and Behaviour," *J R Soc Med.* 1991 December; 84(12): 717–20.

2. The Delta Society lists a variety of studies done to validate the benefits of pet ownership on overall health: **www.deltasociety.org/page.aspx?pid=333**.

Turn on Some Tunes

1. This was obtained on the following website: **www.musictherapy.org**.

Eat Right

1. Miraval's cookbook, *Mindful Eating* (Hay House, 2012), is a great resource for learning healthy and nutritious recipes.

2. True Food Kitchen; go to Fox Restaurant Concepts, **www.foxrc.com**, for restaurant locations.

3. Michael Pollen, *Food Rules* (New York: Penguin Press, 2009).

4. Dr. Andrew Weil (**www.drweil.com**) is famous for his books on the anti-inflammatory diet, including: *Healthy Aging, Eating for Optimum Health, The Healthy Kitchen, Spontaneous Happiness*.

5. Walter C. Willet and P. J. Skerrett, *Eat, Drink and Be Healthy: The Harvard Medical School Guide to Healthy Eating* (New York: Free Press, 2002); Artemis P. Simopaulos and Jo Robinson, *The Omega Diet: The Lifesaving Nutritional Program Based on the Diet of the Island of Crete* (New York: HarperPerrenial, 1999).

6. The British Medical Journal published this meta-analysis on the health benefits of following the Mediterranean Diet: "Adherence to Mediterranean diet and health status: meta-analysis," Francesco Sofi, Francesca Cesari, Rosanna Abbate, Gian Franco Gensini, Alessandro Casini. *BMJ* 2008; 337:a1344, Published 11 September 2008. doi: 10.1136/bmj.a1344.

Use Olive Oil Abundantly

1. This comes from the following article by Beauchamp and others entitled: "Phytochemistry: ibuprofen-like activity in extra-virgin olive oil" in the September, 2005 edition of Nature, 437 (7055): 45–6. New research appearing in a recent arthritis journal suggests oleocanthol's anti-inflammatory effects

on cartilage in an animal model: "Effect of oleocanthal and its derivatives on inflammatory response induced by lipopolysaccharide in a murine chondrocyte cell line." *Arthritis Rheumatology.* 2010 Jun;62(6): 1675–82.

Develop a Taste for Tea

1. H. N. Graham, "Green tea Composition, Consumption, and Polyphenol Chemistry,: *Preventative Medicine* 21 (1992): 334–50; K. Imai and K. Nakachi, "Cross Sectional Study of Effects of Drinking Green Tea on Cardiovascular and Liver Diseases," *British Medical Journal* 310 (1995): 693–96; W. Zheng et al, "Tea Consumption and Cancer Incidence in a Prospective Cohort Study of Postmenopausal Women," *American Journal of Epidemiology* 144 (1996): 175–82; Drug Discovery Program, Biosciences Division, SRI International, "Green Tea and Its Polyphenolic Catechins: Medicinal Uses in Cancer and Noncancer Applications," *Life Sciences* 27;78 (18) March 2006: 2073–80.

2. North Shore-Long Island Jewish Health System (2007, November 8). "EGCG in Green Tea Is Powerful Medicine Against Severe Sepsis, Lab Study Suggests." *Science Daily.*

3. Leone M., Zhai D., Sareth S., Kitada S, Reed J. C., Pellecchia M. (December 2003). "Cancer prevention by tea polyphenols is linked to their direct inhibition of antiapoptotic Bcl-2-family proteins." Cancer Research 63 (23): 8118–21.

My Favorite Breakfast

1. E. J. Stevenson et al. "Oxidation during Exercise and Satiety during Recovery Are increased following a Low-Glycemic Index Breakfast in Sedentary Women." *J. Nutr.* May, 2009 139:5 890–97.

Lay Off the Processed Stuff

1. The glycemic index of common carbohydrate foods are derived from K. Foster-Powell and J.B. Miller, "International Tables of Glycemic Index," *American Journal of Clinical Nutrition* 62 (1995): 871S–93S; Walter Willet, JoAnn Manson, Simin Liu, "Glycemic Index, Glycemic Load and Risk of Type II Diabetes," *American Journal of Clinical Nutrition* 76 (July 2002): 274S–80S.

Practice Hari Hachi Bu

1. Bradley J. Wilcox, D. Craig Wilcox, and Makota Suzuki, *The Okinawa Program: How the World's Longest-Lived People Achieve Everlasting Health—and How You Can Too* (New York: Three Rivers Press, 2002).

"Bate, Bate Chocolate"

1.   You can learn more about the song and the *mulinillo* on the following website: **www.gourmetsleuth.com.**

2.   Zubaida Faridi et al. "Acute dark chocolate and cocoa ingestion and endothelial function: a randomized controlled crossover trial," *American Journal of Clinical Nutrition,* Vol. 88, No. 1, 58–63, July 2008. Triche, EW, et al. "Chocolate consumption in pregnancy and reduced likelihood of preeclampsia," *Epidemiology,* May 19, 2008 (3): 459–64. Taubert, D. *The Journal of the American Medical Association,* Aug. 27, 2003; vol 290: 1029–30. Serafini, M. *Nature,* Aug. 28, 2003; vol 424: 1013. U.S. Department of Agriculture Nutrient Data Laboratory. Penny M. Kris-Etherton and Vikkie A. Mustad, "Chocolate Feeding Studies: A Novel Approach for Evaluating the Plasma Lipid Effects of Stearic Acid," *American Journal of Clinical Nutrition* 60 (6 supplement), 1029S–36S, 1994.

Drink More Water

1.   Rose BD et al. "Maintenance and replacement fluid therapy in adults." **http:// www.uptodate.com/home/index.html**; "Dietary reference intakes for water, potassium, sodium, chloride and sulfate." Institute of Medicine. **www.nal .usda.gov/fnic/DRI//DRI_Water/73-185.pdf**; Exercise and fluid replacement. *Medicine & Science in Sports & Exercise.* 2007;39:377; Campbell SM. "Hydration needs throughout the lifespan." *American Journal of Clinical Nutrition.* 2007; 26:585S; "Nutrition and athletic performance: Position of the American Dietetic Association, Dietitians of Canada, and the American College of Sports Medicine." *Journal of the American Dietetic Association.* 2009; 109:509. Howard Murad, *The Water Secret* (Hoboken, NJ: Wiley, 2010).

Optimize Your Vitamin D

1.   Much of the research I have gathered has come from Dr. Michael Holick, either in the form of his website—**www.vitamindhealth.org**—or his recent book: *The Vitamin D Solution: A 3-Step Strategy to Cure Our Most Common Health Problem* (New York: Hudson Street Press, 2010).

Take a Good Daily Multivitamin-Mineral Supplement

1.   David F. Horrobin, "Food, Micronutrients, and Psychiatry," *Int Psychogeriat* 14 no.4 (January 2005): 331–34.

Get More Omega-3s

1. Cynthia Graber, "Snake Oil Salesmen Were on to Something," *Scientific American,* November, 1, 2007. Richard Kunin, "Snake Oil," *Western Journal of Medicine,* 151 no.2 (August 1989): 208.

2. Bunea R., El Ferrah K., Deutsch, L. "Evaluation of the Effects of Neptune Krill Oil on the Clinical Course of Hyperlipidemia," *Altern Med Rev 9,* 4 (2004): 420–28. Deutsch, L. "Evaluation of the Effect of Neptune Krill Oil on Chronic Inflammation and Arthritic Symptoms," *Journal of the American College of Nutrition,* 26 1 (2007): 39–48.

3. T. A. Mori, et al. "Effects of Varying Dietary Fat, Fish and Fish Oils on Blood Lipids in a Randomized Controlled Trial in Men at Risk of Heart Disease," *American Journal of Clinical Nutrition* 59 (1994): 4160–69; Pauletto, "Blood Pressure and Atherogenic Lipoprotein Profiles in Fish-Diet and Vegetarian Villagers in Tanzania: The Lugawala Study," *Lancet* 348 (1996): 784–88; GISSI-Prevenzione Investigators, Dietary Supplements with n-3 Poly-unsaturated Fatty Acids and Vitamin E After Myocardial Infarction: Results of the GISSI-Prevenzioni Trial," *Lancet* 354 (August 1999): 447–55. Artemis Simopaulos, "Omega-3 Fatty Acids in Inflammation and Autoimmune Diseases," *Journal of the American College of Nutrition* 21 (2002): 495–505.

The Magic of Tulsi

1. S. Singh et al. "Evaluation of Anti-inflammatory Potential of Fixed Oil of *Ocimum sanctum* (Holy Basil) and Its Possible Mechanism of Action," *J Ethnopharmacol 54* (1996): 19–26; See also David Winston and Steven Maimes, *Adaptogens: Herbs for Strength, Stamina and Stress relief* (Rochester, VT: Inner Traditions—Bear & Co, 2007); and Dr. Narendra Singh and Dr. Yamuna Hoette, *Tulsi—Mother Medicine of Nature,* International Institute of Herbal Medicine (Lucknow, India), 2002, **www .holybasil.com/6685.html**.

Learn More about 'Shrooms

1. H. Nanba, "Activity of Maitake D-Fraction to Inhibit Carcinogenesis and Metastasis," *Annals of the New York Academy of Sciences* 768 (1995): 243–45; Shah SK, et al., "An evidence-based review of a Lentinula edodes mushroom extract as complementary therapy in the surgical oncology patient." *Journal of Parenteral and Enteral Nutrition* 35 no.4 (2011): 449–58. Yu CH, et al. "Inhibitory mechanisms of Agaricus blazei Murill on the growth of prostate cancer in vitro and in vivo." *J. Nutr. Biochem.* 20 no. 10 (October 2008): 753–64.

2. A. Tsunoo, "*Cordyceps sinensis*: Its Diverse Effects on Mammals in vitro and in vivo," *New Initiatives in Mycological Research,* proceedings of the third International Symposium of the Mycological Society of Japan, Natural History Museum and Institute, Chiba, Japan, 1995; Nicodemus, K. J., et al.,

"Supplementation with Cordyceps Cs-4 fermentation product promotes fat metabolism during prolonged exercise." *Medicine and Science in Sports and Exercise,* 33 (2001): S 164 (Abstract); J. Lin et al., "Radical Scavenger and Antihepatotoxic Activity of *Ganoderma formanosum, Ganoderma lucidum, and Ganoderma neo-japonicum,*" *Journal of Ethnopharmacology* 47 (1995): 33–41.

3. This was taken from the following *NY Times* article that mentioned using winter worm tonics for their athletes. Follow this here: **www.nytimes .com/1994/08/30/sports/swimming-china-is-getting-ready-for-another-big-splash.html?pagewanted=all&src=pm.**

4. **www.powersupplements.com/cordyceps/cordy_article.pdf.**

5. **www.naturalnews.com/027869_cordyceps_cancer.html.**

6. Zhu J. S., Halpern G. M., Jones K. "The scientific rediscovery of a precious ancient Chinese herbal regime: Cordyceps sinensis, *Part I.* " *J Altern Complement Med* 1998; 4: 289–303. Zhu J. S., Halpern G. M., Jones K. "The scientific rediscovery of a precious ancient Chinese herbal regime: Cordyceps sinensis, *Part II.*" *J Altern Complement Med* 1998;4: 429–57.

7. Gao Y., et al. "Effects of Ganopoly (Ganoderma lucidum Polysaccharide Extract) on the Immune Functions in Advanced-Stage Cancer Patients." *Immunol Invest* 2003;32(3): 201–15.

8. Luzio N. R. Williams D. L. et al, "Comparative evaluation of the tumor inhibitory and antibacterial activity of solubilized and particulate glucan," *Recent Results Cancer Res 75: 165–72. 1980.* Okazaki M., Adachi Y., Ohno N., Yadomae T. "Structure-activity relationship of (1Ñ>3)-beta-D-glucans in the induction of cytokine production from macrophages, in vitro." Biol Pharm Bull 1995;18: 1320–7.

9. Mansell P. W., Ichinose H., Reed R. J., et al., "Macrophage-mediated destruction of human malignant cells in vivo," J Natl Cancer Inst. 1975 Mar; 54(3): 571–80. Borchers, A. T.; Krishnamurthy, A.; Keen, C. L.; Meyers, F. J.; Gershwin, M. E. (2008). "The Immunobiology of Mushrooms." Experimental Biology and Medicine 233 (3): 259–76.doi:10.3181/0708-MR-227. PMID 18296732.

10. Paul Stamets is one of the leading mycologists in the world. He is author of several books, including *Mycelium Running: How Mushrooms Can Help Save the World* (Berkeley, CA: Ten Speed Press, 2005). Learn more about the medicinal aspects of mushrooms on his website: **www.fungi.com.**

Walk the Dog

1. See the following website from the Delta Society and from the CDC: **www.cdc .gov/healthypets/health_benefits.htm.**

2. Dennis Thompson Jr., "Pet therapy and Depression," *Everyday Health,* 2011. Edney ATB, "Companion Animals and Human Health: An Overview," *Journal of the Royal Society of Medicine* 88 (1995):704P–8P.

3. The Harvard Alumni Study is a prospective observational study of approximately 17,000 men who attended Harvard between 1916 and 1950. The results of a 16-year follow up of physical activity levels and all causes of mortality showed that greater levels of exercise were associated with lower risk of death of all causes. Expending just 500 to 900 extra calories per week in physical activity significantly reduced the relative risk of mortality by greater than 20 percent. For further information, refer to the following citation: Paffenbarger R. S. Jr., Hyde R. T., Wing A. L., Hsieh C. C. "Physical Activity, All-Cause Mortality and Longevity of College Alumni," *N Engl J Med,* 1986 Mar 6;314(10): 605–13.

Move Your Body Every Day

1. Denise Milton et al., "The Effect of Functional Exercise Training on Functional Fitness Levels of Older Adults," *Gundersen Lutheran Medical Journal,* Volume 5, Number 1 (July 2008): 4–8; Nieman DC, et al., "The immune response to a 30-minute walk," *Med Sci Sports Exerc* 37 (2005): 57–62; How much exercise do you need? **http://www.cdc.gov/nccdphp/dnpa/physical/everyone/ recommendations/index.htm.**

   Exercise: How much is enough? ClevelandClinic: **http://my.clevelandclinic. org/heart/prevention/exercise/howmuchisenough.aspx.**

High-Intensity Interval Training

1. Trembblay, A., Simoneau, J. A., Bouchard C., "Impact of Exercise Intensity on Body Fatness and Skeletal Muscle Metabolism," *Metabolism,* 43 no7 (1994): 814–18.

Strength Training

1. Available in the form of a fact sheet that you can download from their website titled, "Exercise Is Medicine": **http://exerciseismedicine.org/documents/ EIMFactSheet2012_all.pdf.**

2. For reference, there are great videos and diagrams to show the various weight-lifting exercises to try. Get on the Body for Life website or Bill Phillips's home page: **www.transformation.com.**

Know Your Trigger Points

1. Doctors Janet Travell and David Simons; their work is in a two-volume medical textbook entitled *Myofascial Pain and Dysfunction: The Trigger Point Manual.* (Lippincott, Williams & Wilkins, 1992).

Afterword

1. Dr. Andrew Weil, *8 Weeks to Optimum Health,* **www.drweil.com**.

2. William Goldman, *The Princess Bride* (New York: Ballantine Books, 2003).

ACKNOWLEDGMENTS

A number of people have helped me write this book. Some of you know how much you've contributed, whereas others may not.

Knowing that this is my first venture into the literary world, I would like to begin by offering thanks to my parents, Adeo and Barbara Nicolai. From an early age, you instilled in me a deep passion for knowledge from people and books, movies and music, and the adventure that goes with them. I am eternally grateful for your inspiration. Thanks also go out to my brother, Michael. You are the Fratello Straordinario. *Multi grazii* for always being there, no matter what.

Thanks so much to everyone at Miraval who gave me a chance to live my dream, from Michael Tompkins, who gave me my first job here; to all of the experts and practitioners who have inspired me with their knowledge and skill. To Junelle Lupiani—dietician extraordinaire; Andrew Wolf—perhaps the smartest man I know, and a darn good botanist to boot; and Anne Parker—the work we did together was life-changing and continues to keeps me on task. Thank you for your insight. I need to also thank Mark Pirtle, whose vision for healing is a mirror of my own. I relish our talks. Coach Leigh, you are a force of nature that cannot be contained. Your *joie de vivre* is infectious, and you challenge others to find their bliss. Rock on, sister! Experiencing Chi Nei Tsang and craniosacral therapy from Lolita and Tama was powerful; the effects of your work were not subtle. Neither was deep tissue work with Manny or Spirit Flight from Dr. Tim Frank, whose skillful ceremony and hands made me soar to a wonderful place. I appreciate your challenge, Tim, for both of us to be the best healers possible.

My relationship with Dr. Andrew Weil goes beyond words. You have been more than a mentor and friend. I feel that our brotherhood suspends time and distance. I am glad to be closer to home. Thanks also to Richard Baxter, who has always offered me great advice and words straight from the heart. I always appreciate your honesty and candor. Hopefully, the Colts can be good again.

Many authors have inspired me along the way. Their work has bled into mine, and if I have forgotten to mention them properly, it was not intentional. Specifically, I need to give a special thanks to Steven Pressfield. First off, I'm a big fan. You turned me on to ancient Greece before I ever thought about doing "the work." More important, your recent books have challenged me to enter the literary bullring and start waving my *muleta*. Thanks for your guidance along the way. I've still got my head down, looking for the guy who's trying to poke me in the butt. As the Spartans say, "Do not ask how many are the enemy but where they are!" Thanks for showing me that sometimes the enemy is staring me in the face, and he is me.

To the folks at Hay House, thanks for giving me the opportunity to be a writer. You are the ultimate professionals; and with your guidance, wisdom, and gentle nudges, you made this book a better one. A big shout-out also has to go to editor extraordinaire Cyndy Neighbors. You and your team at Many Hats went above and beyond the call of duty. Cyndy, you challenged me to improve as a writer. Thank you so much; all of your suggestions were spot-on.

I also owe an amazing debt to the thousands of clients I have seen, taught, and had the great honor of working with through more than ten years as a practicing physician. You have taught me patience, humility, compassion, and resilience. I have learned that the beauty of medicine is expressed fully when I get a chance to hear another person's story—who you are, what you've done, what's gotten you to this place in your life, and where you might want to go if that destination isn't ideal. Your stories have enriched my life and made me realize what an incredible gift it is to be a doctor. Helping others get closer to health and wellness is a privilege. You've stretched me beyond my limits and made me the physician I am today. I hope to be challenged by the stories you continue to offer me.

Finally, I want to say thanks to my kids, Kyle, Jude, and Ava, for always keeping me busy and smiling (for the most part, anyway). Family is truly everything to me; without it, I am nothing. In addition, my wife, Sara, has been amazing during this project. She has suffered through endless drafts of this book and inarguably been my best proofreader. She dots the I's and crosses the T's better than anyone. More than that, Sara, you have offered amazing ideas and health tips that wouldn't have been in this book if not for your creativity and insight. I mention you in these pages because you are such an important piece of my life and what I do to stay healthy. You are my perfect counterpart, Sara Sue. I love you lots.

And ultimately, I couldn't end this book without thanking my Creator, who has blessed me with guidance, inspiration, and an absolute feeling of clarity—that I was on the right path—throughout this entire process. You are good all the time, and I am grateful. And thanks for the hawk fly-bys (my spiritual totem). It's nice to know you're out there.

ABOUT THE AUTHOR

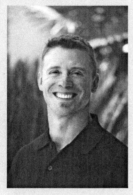

James P. Nicolai, MD, is the medical director of the Andrew Weil, MD, Integrative Wellness Program at Miraval Resort and Spa, the first interactive integrative wellness programme of its kind at a destination spa resort. He is a board-certified family practitioner and a graduate of the Integrative Medicine Fellowship at the University of Arizona in Tucson, under the direction of Dr Andrew Weil. A graduate of the Indiana School of Medicine, Dr Nicolai completed his family practice residency at St. Francis Hospital and Health Centers.

Dr Nicolai has a special interest in whole-person medicine, addressing patients as mental and emotional beings, energetic and spiritual entities and community members, as well as physical bodies. His expertise is in combining conventional medicine with the intelligent use of complementary and alternative therapies, including herbs and other botanicals, vitamins and supplements, nutritional counselling, lifestyle management and stress reduction.

www.drjimnicolai.com

NOTES

NOTES

We hope you enjoyed this Hay House book. If you'd like
to receive our online catalogue featuring additional information on
Hay House books and products, or if you'd like to find out
more about the Hay Foundation, please contact:

Hay House UK, Ltd., 292B Kensal Rd., London W10 5BE
Phone: 0-20-8962-1230 • *Fax:* 0-20-8962-1239
www.hayhouse.co.uk • **www.hayfoundation.org**

Published and distributed in the United States by:
Hay House, Inc., P.O. Box 5100, Carlsbad, CA 92018-5100
Phone: (760) 431-7695 or (800) 654-5126 or
Fax: (760) 431-6948 or (800) 650-5115
www.hayhouse.com®

Published and distributed in Australia by: Hay House Australia Pty. Ltd.,
18/36 Ralph St., Alexandria NSW 2015 • *Phone:* 612-9669-4299
Fax: 612-9669-4144 • www.hayhouse.com.au

Published and distributed in the Republic of South Africa by: Hay House SA (Pty),
Ltd., P.O. Box 990, Witkoppen 2068 • *Phone/Fax:* 27-11-467-8904
www.hayhouse.co.za

Published in India by: Hay House Publishers India, Muskaan Complex,
Plot No. 3, B-2, Vasant Kunj, New Delhi 110 070 • *Phone:* 91-11-4176-1620
Fax: 91-11-4176-1630 • www.hayhouse.co.in

Distributed in Canada by: Raincoast, 9050 Shaughnessy St., Vancouver, B.C.
V6P 6E5 • *Phone:* (604) 323-7100 • *Fax:* (604) 323-2600 • www.raincoast.com

Take Your Soul on a Vacation

Visit **www.HealYourLife.com**® to regroup, recharge,
and reconnect with your own magnificence.
Featuring blogs, mind-body-spirit news, and life-changing
wisdom from Louise Hay and friends.

Visit **www.HealYourLife.com** today!

Free e-newsletters
from Hay House, the Ultimate
Resource for Inspiration

Be the first to know about Hay House's dollar deals, free downloads, special offers, affirmation cards, giveaways, contests, and more!

 Get exclusive excerpts from our latest releases and videos from *Hay House Present Moments*.

 Enjoy uplifting personal stories, how-to articles, and healing advice, along with videos and empowering quotes, within *Heal Your Life*.

 Have an inspirational story to tell and a passion for writing? Sharpen your writing skills with insider tips from *Your Writing Life*.

Sign Up Now!

Get inspired, educate yourself, get a complimentary gift, and share the wisdom!

http://www.hayhouse.com/newsletters.php

Visit www.hayhouse.com to sign up today!

HealYourLife.com

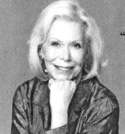
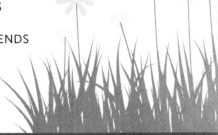

JOIN THE HAY HOUSE FAMILY

As the leading self-help, mind, body and spirit publisher in the UK, we'd like to welcome you to our family so that you can enjoy all the benefits our website has to offer.

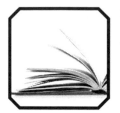 **EXTRACTS** from a selection of your favourite author titles

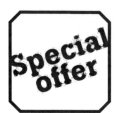 **COMPETITIONS, PRIZES & SPECIAL OFFERS** Win extracts, money off, downloads and so much more

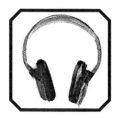 **LISTEN** to a range of radio interviews and our latest audio publications

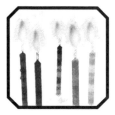 **CELEBRATE YOUR BIRTHDAY** An inspiring gift will be sent your way

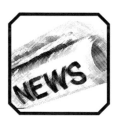 **LATEST NEWS** Keep up with the latest news from and about our authors

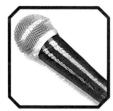 **ATTEND OUR AUTHOR EVENTS** Be the first to hear about our author events

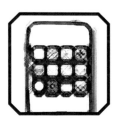 **iPHONE APPS** Download your favourite app for your iPhone

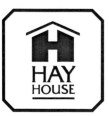 **HAY HOUSE INFORMATION** Ask us anything, all enquiries answered

join us online at **www.hayhouse.co.uk**

 292B Kensal Road, London W10 5BE
T: 020 8962 1230 E: info@hayhouse.co.uk